ETHICS

EDUCATION
AND RESEARCH

Edited by

Verena Tschudin BSc (Hons), RGN, RM,
Dip Counselling

Illustrations by Richard Smith

Scutari Press · London

A division of Scutari Projects Ltd, the publishing company of the Royal College of Nursing

First published 1994

British Library Cataloguing in Publication Data
Education and Research. – (Ethics Series)
  I. Tschudin, Verena   II. Series
  170
   ISBN 1–873853–11–4

Phototypeset by Intype, London
Printed and bound in Great Britain by
Athenæum Press Ltd, Gateshead, Tyne & Wear.

Contents

Contents

Contributors

Gillian Little RGN, RM, JBCNS

Clinical Nurse Specialist, Stoma Care, Basildon and Thurrock General Hospitals Trust

Diane Marks-Maran BSc, RGN, DipN (Lond), RNT

Director, Academic Development Department, Queen Charlotte's College, London

Barbara Parker

Secretary to the Board, Royal Marsden NHS Trust

Win Tadd BEd (Hons), RGN, RM, DipN (Lond), ONC, RCNT, RNT

Senior Teacher, South East Wales Institute of Nursing and Midwifery Education

Preface

Ethics is not only at the heart of nursing, it *is* the heart of nursing. Ethics is about what is right and good. Nursing and caring are synonymous, and the way in which care is carried out is ethically decisive. How a patient is addressed, cared for and treated must be right not only by ordinary standards of care, but also by ethical principles.

These ethical principles have not always been addressed clearly, but now patients, nurses, doctors and all types of health care personnel are questioning their care in the light of ethics. Their starting points and approaches are different, but their 'results' are remarkably similar. The individual person matters and the care given and received has to be human and humanising.

The way in which the contributors to this volume, and others in the series, address their subject is also individual and unique. Their brief was simply that what they wrote should be applicable to practising nurses. Each chapter reflects the personal style and approach of the writer. This is what gives this series its distinctive character and strength, and provides the reader with the opportunity to see different approaches working. It is hoped that this will encourage readers to think that their own way of understanding ethics and behaving ethically is also acceptable and worthwhile. Theories and principles are important, and so are their interpretation and application. That is a job for everybody, not just the experts: experts can point the way — as in this series of books — but all nurses need to be challenged and encouraged.

Emphasis is laid in all the chapters on the individual nurse and patient or client. Ethics 'happens' between and among people, and, by the authors bringing their own experience to bear on their chapters, they show how ethics works in relationships.

Great achievements often start with a small idea quite different from the end result, and so it is with this series of books. The initial proposal is almost unrecognisable in the final product. Many people contributed to the growth of the idea, many more were involved in implementing it, and I hope that even more will benefit from it.

My particular thanks go to Geoff Hunt, Director of the European Centre for Professional Ethics, University of East London, for his advice and help with this series.

Verena Tschudin

CHAPTER 1

Ethics in the Curriculum

Win Tadd

'Seeing with a moral eye' would have been on Florence
Nightingale's curriculum had she thought of the expression
and considered it necessary to teach the subject. Ethics has
always been implicit in nursing, but only recently has it
become important enough to be considered a topic for
teaching.

For nurse teachers who may not know what and how to teach
in ethics, this chapter gives some very clear guidelines and
insights. All readers, whether teachers or those who are taught,
will gain from this chapter and the insights it offers into
approaches to caring which are stimulating and 'holistic'.

Considering that nursing is so closely involved with human
suffering and human nurturing, it is undoubtedly a great
indictment of nurse education that, until quite recently,
ethics teaching has had a very low profile in schools and
colleges of nursing in the UK. Over the past 20 or 30
years, there has been an increasing focus on the topic of
ethics education in the nursing literature, although this has
been almost exclusively American in origin.

The impetus to incorporate formal ethics education in
nursing courses at both pre- and post-registration levels is
the result of a number of recent developments. One of the
most important of these has been the requirement of
the UKCC that courses leading to registration now require
'an understanding of the ethics of health care and of the
nursing profession and the responsibilities which these
impose on the nurse's professional practice' (Statutory
Instruments 1989). There are, however, other factors

which account for the explosion of interest in nursing ethics.

The first of these is the increasing public and professional realisation that central to many of the developments and advances in health care are questions relating to moral choice and individual and societal values.

Secondly, technological advances have pushed forward the frontiers of possibility at an alarming rate, creating greater public expectations of both treatment choices and outcomes. These advances have great implications for the practice of all health care professionals, particularly for nurses, who spend most time in close proximity to clients and their families.

Thirdly, despite technological advancement, the resources available for health care remain finite at both the macro and micro levels of health care provision. At the macro level, policy decisions are made not only about which treatment choices will be offered, but also in relation to which groups should benefit. For instance, in vitro fertilisation is now more widely available in society generally, but it is currently not considered a suitable intervention for those individuals who are mildly mentally handicapped and wishing to become parents.

At the micro level, it is often the nurse who is faced with the consequences of such policy decisions. For example, the decision to reduce the number of hip replacement operations or the number of heart transplants affects the nature of nurses' work, just as efficiency savings within the local hospital affect the resources they have at their disposal for day-to-day care.

Fourthly, the current political ideologies emphasising consumer choice, rights and individualism have forced all professional groups to reconsider their relationship with their clients.

Fifthly, the increasing emphasis on advocacy, accountability and responsibility has forced nurses to consider the nature of their association with clients, co-workers and employing institutions. This is evidenced by the formulation and publication of documents such as the *Code of Professional Conduct* (UKCC 1983, 1984, 1992a), and *Exercising Accountability* (UKCC 1989). These have all highlighted the possible conflicts which ensue when nurses are expected to function as independent professionals within a bureaucratic system.

Finally, and perhaps most importantly, there are signs that nursing is at last coming of age in the UK. With this has come a recognition of the importance of making explicit a nursing philosophy and an ethic that emphasises the centrality of the client and the importance of care as opposed to cure, along with the need to humanise the patient's experience of health care, especially when all other emphasis appears to be on throughput and outcomes. This has resulted in the realisation by nurses themselves that an understanding of the humanities generally, and ethics in particular, can be of real value in the clinical situation. Perhaps it is this dawning that has led to the greatest demand for ethics to be a formal part of nurses' education.

Issues in Ethics Education

The inclusion of ethics in the nursing curriculum raises a number of issues and questions which will be explored in this chapter. These include:

- the aims of ethics education;
- how ethics might be incorporated into the curriculum;
- what might count as appropriate content;
- how and by whom this content should be taught;
- how learning might be assessed;

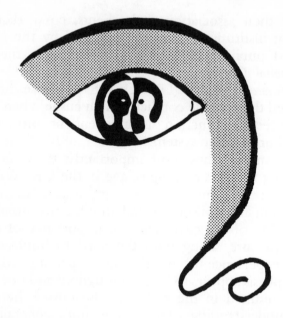

- what implications might result from the introduction of ethics into programmes of nurse education.

The emphasis will be on assisting those who are charged with the responsibility of implementing such a course to think about the problems and practicalities of this task.

Until quite recently, there has been relatively little guidance in British literature to help and advise those wishing to incorporate philosophy and/or ethics into programmes of nurse education (see Further Reading, below). One particularly useful text is a work based on the results of a study of ethics teaching in nursing spanning the whole of the UK (Gallagher and Boyd, 1991). In the course of their research, Gallagher and Boyd discovered that despite a great deal of interest in the topic, aims, when articulated, were often incompatible, content was not clearly identified, teachers were rarely prepared for such teaching, and when taught, ethics content was rarely assessed. It is hoped that this chapter will make a positive contribution to rectifying this situation.

Before commencing on a discussion of the issues listed above, it may be useful to define some of the terms which are frequently referred to in the literature and which may be confusing to those who are not familiar with the subject area.

Commonly, ethics is defined as the study of the nature and grounds of morality, where morality is taken as the general term for the judgements, standards and rules governing how one behaves towards others. It therefore involves exploring concepts such as right and wrong and good and bad. In philosophy, ethics is often divided into three branches: descriptive ethics, metaethics and normative ethics.

Descriptive ethics, as the name implies, offers an objective account of the moral behaviour, attitudes or beliefs of particular persons, groups or societies. Metaethics is concerned with three basic tasks (Taylor, 1975):

- analysing the meaning of terms used in moral discourse, such as right or good;
- examining the logic or reasoning of moral discourse;
- considering how the truth or otherwise of moral beliefs or claims can be known.

Normative ethics involves prescribing norms or standards of behaviour or conduct and, as such, explores moral arguments and actions in such a way as to determine what is good or bad, praiseworthy or blameworthy, and which ends or circumstances ought to be furthered in society. It is largely with the teaching of normative ethics that this chapter will deal.

Within the category of normative ethics, a further subcategory is currently enjoying an increasing emphasis and popularity, namely that of applied ethics. This is evidenced by the growing numbers of postgraduate programmes in topics such as social ethics, bioethics, and health care ethics. Applied ethics is the term used when ethical or moral enquiry is focused on concrete moral problems and conflicts to enable practical moral decision-making. Professional ethics is an aspect or area of applied ethics that is specifically concerned with studying the moral or ethical dimension of professional conduct, both in general terms and in relation to specific occupational or professional groups. Nursing ethics, medical ethics and business ethics are all examples of areas covered by professional ethics.

Having clarified some of the terminology, attention can now be given to the specific issues involved with the inclusion of ethics in the nursing curriculum.

The Aims of Ethics Teaching

The purpose of moral education has been the subject of a long-standing debate in the philosophy of education and will largely remain so as far as this text is concerned, as it is assumed that a knowledge of ethics constitutes an important element of the nurse's professional preparation. It is important, however, that those wishing to introduce the subject of ethics into a nursing course should make their motives for such a decision clear. Not only is such an activity more likely to lead to the identification and inclusion of appropriate content, to course processes and to the ability to evaluate how successful one has been, but it will also reduce the potential for suspicion which can be found in certain quarters when such additions to the educational programme are suggested. The six aims discussed below are not intended to be an exhaustive list; instead they serve to indicate important areas that deserve consideration.

Developing moral consciousness

A fundamental aspect of any course in ethics should be to ensure that students appreciate that, rather than it being a sterile academic exercise, there are significant practical consequences of all moral deliberation. As Strawson (1982) makes clear, people everywhere live their lives within a 'general structure or web of human attitudes and feelings' and it is that complicated web of feelings, attitudes and relationships 'which forms an essential part of the moral life as we know it'.

It is vital, therefore, that students gain a feel for the impact of various moral positions or rules on the lives of other people and the resultant misery or pleasure which different ethical choices can bring. Helping students to realise this should be a key outcome in relation to this aim. Students also need to appreciate that it is largely individuals' moral standpoints that influence how they live their lives and relate to others.

In addition, it is necessary to emphasise that moral conflicts and dilemmas are often an unavoidable aspect of human life, let alone nursing practice, and also that they are notoriously difficult to resolve. An acceptance of this will help students to see that they are not unique and that they share the common problem of facing and coping with moral conflict. As nurses, however, their decisions and actions affect the most vulnerable members of society, so how they deal with moral conflicts and dilemmas assumes an even greater importance than for the man or woman 'in the street'.

Students should also be prepared to face the range and strength of the negative and positive feelings that moral considerations can evoke and the role that they may play in determining their moral actions. Feelings such as empathy, guilt, repugnance, care, sympathy, pity, sadness or outrage can be very powerful emotions, and students need to recognise that such feelings may change considerably after a more detailed analysis of a particular situation has been undertaken. From this, students learn that although their initial reaction may be correct, it can never be merely assumed or taken for granted. Feelings are not necessarily indicators of what is right or wrong or, indeed, good or evil.

Seeing with a moral eye

A natural progression from developing a moral conscious-ness is assisting students to 'see with a moral eye', so that they can detect and identify the ethical dimensions and issues in their day-to-day work. For a profession that prides itself on its practitioners' powers of observation, this element of nurses' education has in the past been sadly ignored, if not actively discouraged. No doubt many nurses have undergone a professional preparation that proclaimed the wisdom of remaining distant and aloof, and of not allowing oneself to become emotionally involved with patients and clients. Thankfully, a different message is being transmitted today as the concept of care becomes an auth-entic area for academic focus.

A vital ingredient of an ethic of care is a commitment to the one cared for (Noddings, 1984). Part of this com-mitment involves seeing in a moral sense as embraced by Iris Murdoch (1970) in *The Sovereignty of Good*, when she states that 'clear vision is a result of moral imagination and moral effort'. For Murdoch, 'moral looking' becomes a habit which 'goes on continually' rather than being 'some-thing that is switched off in between the occurrence of moral choices'.

This is an important idea for students to grasp, as all too frequently in discussion with nurses the assumption is that ethics is concerned only with momentous decisions such as those involved in euthanasia, abortion or withdrawing life-saving treatments. It is important for nursing students to recognise that ethics is part and parcel of everyday nursing activities. Geoff Hunt gives a wonderful example of the ordinariness of moral activity in his criticism of a nurse writing in a prominent nursing journal who recommends that clients in intensive care units should have a window, a clock, periods of undisturbed sleep and someone to talk to, to avoid sensory imbalance and behavioural disturbances. As Hunt points out, scientific reasoning and rationales are not necessary to justify these amenities; simple human decency and moral common sense are reason enough (Hunt, 1991).

Nurses also need to be aware that it is very easy to reduce moral decisions to clinical ones. For example, the decision to keep an unfavourable prognosis from a patient, without first ascertaining the patient's wishes, is in fact an ethical decision rather than a clinical one. Yet all too often, even senior nurses accept the clinical authority of the doctor to make such decisions, frequently agreeing to lie to patients, rather than challenging the doctor's right unilaterally to make such a judgement in the first place. Failure to question such abuse of authority and to promote team discussion, rather than accept the decisions of others as absolute, robs individual clients of the opportunity to be in control of their lives. It also treats nurses as objects or instruments who are there simply to carry out orders and act on instructions, regardless of the consequences for themselves or others.

The ability to discern when issues are of a moral nature, to spot implicit value positions and to appreciate the implications of decisions are therefore cardinal ends to be promoted in the education of nurses.

Developing skills in critical thinking

Developing the students' skills in critical thinking has been an educational aim which has been popular since the origins of Western philosophy in ancient Greece, and although all teachers can claim that their role involves achieving this aim, a particular emphasis is placed on these skills in ethics teaching. Undoubtedly, this is in part due to ethics being a branch of philosophy, a subject in which logic and reasoning are traditional tools. The word 'critical' has its roots in the Latin 'criticus', meaning a judge or decision-maker. For ethics to have practical value, students need to be able to discern when issues are of a moral nature. This depends on their understanding of various moral concepts such as rights, freedom, autonomy and respect, along with their ability to analyse what is involved in the application of such complex and abstract notions to their daily practice.

Critical thinking involves more than grasping rudimentary notions of logic, blueprints for problem-solving or, indeed, learning definitions of complex concepts. It also requires that students engage in what Dewey (1910) referred to as 'reflective thought', which involves a willingness to suspend judgement, to maintain a healthy scepticism and to exercise an open mind. How this aim might be achieved will be explored in greater detail when specific content and teaching and learning methods are examined.

Accepting dissension and clarifying meanings

The very nature of ethics is such that the likelihood of disagreement on specific issues is great, even with those who are closest, let alone acquaintances or professional colleagues. Furthermore, with many ethical issues, there can be no single or crystal clear solution. Despite the fact that ultimate moral judgements will always be an individual concern, ethics is not simply a matter of personal opinion, and students need help to come to terms with the frustrations that this factor necessarily raises. A very useful account of this problem can be found in *Challenges in Caring* by Brown, Kitson and McKnight (1992).

A course in ethics should encourage students to pinpoint and elucidate any sources of disagreement, an activity which frequently involves clarifying not only the meanings of specific terms, but also the ways in which they are used. Within this subject, the potential for ambiguity and speaking at cross-purposes is great. Although every individual is her or his own moral authority, it is as sagacious in ethics as it is in other areas of decision-making to consider a wide range of views before reaching an ultimate conclusion.

Encouraging an awareness of moral responsibility

Because people are their own moral authority, it is important that individuals appreciate that this demands accepting responsibility for their own moral decisions and judgements. Excuses such as 'I was merely following orders' or 'My hands are clean, I didn't get involved' are rarely acceptable in judging the consequences of moral behaviour. Morality not only involves an agent's direct actions, but also her or his omissions and responsibility, as these cannot be parcelled up and passed along the line because they are inconvenient to retain.

With nursing's tradition of obedience and subservience, as well as its hierarchical structure, it is particularly important that novice nurses acquire this sense of moral obligation and responsibility. This inevitably leads to discussions of freedom and the role of freedom in moral agency. Similarly, in relation to promoting a sense of moral obligation, the teacher cannot escape addressing questions of why one should be moral and what it means to be so. The potential minefields which any teacher may unwittingly walk into when discussing these topics will be considered later.

Promoting moral behaviour

This is perhaps the most contentious of all the aims so far discussed, and some readers may well disagree that this should be an explicit intention of an ethics course. Others may feel that it is somewhat naïve to believe that students will in fact modify their behaviour as a direct result of any teaching. The latter criticism may well be true, but surely the ultimate aim of all education is that students will learn and that, as a result of that learning, their behaviour will change.

One of the reasons behind the denial of this as a legitimate goal of moral education is the justifiable fear that this aim may result in the use of very questionable teaching methods that involve the manipulation and indoctrination of students. The validity of such a fear depends to a very large extent on how the term 'moral behaviour' is defined. If by this term is meant transmitting preordained moral conclusions on how students ought to respond in various situations and how they ought to define what is in fact moral or ethical in specific instances, these objections would be well-founded.

There is, however, an alternative definition of 'moral behaviour', which provides a wholly worthwhile aim of ethics teaching. This would involve developing in students the ability and willingness to engage in self-analysis and self-criticism when reflecting on their own moral positions and actions, as well as a preparedness to change if this is indicated by such reflection. In addition, a willingness publicly to justify and explain how and why a particular position is held, or certain actions are performed or omitted, is an important aspect of accepting both moral and professional responsibility.

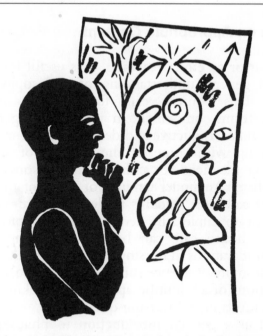

It might, indeed, be argued that it is futile to cultivate the ability to perceive moral issues, reason ethically and listen to and respect the viewpoints of others, if one does not intend that students will in fact utilise these skills in their clinical practice. It is in these ways that students should be encouraged and assisted to behave morally.

Finally, there is always the danger that students will simply use their newly-acquired skills to defend obviously questionable moral positions and to demonstrate thinly veiled sophistry. It is essential, therefore, that the importance of moral consciousness and the consequences of ignoring moral considerations in nursing are emphasised. By doing this, every student should be aware of how nursing itself is an ethical or moral endeavour, which has as its ultimate aim the humanising of health care and the maximisation of human potential (Seedhouse, 1988).

Deciding on Appropriate Content

As a precursor to ethics teaching, it is useful for students to have a general understanding of philosophy and its methods. This content can, for example, introduce important terms, on which an understanding of ethics frequently relies. Inductive and deductive reasoning can be taught, along with some of the fallacies of argument, emphasising the need for coherence and consistency in ethical debate. An understanding of different theories of knowledge can assist students in developing an awareness of how, for example, the technorational approaches to health and health care can have a direct impact upon ethical considerations in nursing. Similarly, an introduction to the philosophy of science can help students to appreciate the limitations of a scientific approach in seeking answers to certain fundamental nursing questions.

As well as a general introduction to philosophy, the topic of values education also needs to be addressed. Undoubtedly, one of the factors which most affects the decisions that individuals make are the values that they hold in relation to themselves and others and how they view the world generally. Once individuals can identify, clarify and analyse their own values and appreciate the role that they play in shaping their decisions and behaviour, they will be able to acquire a clearer understanding of ethics, along with the ability to make and accept the consequences of their ethical decisions.

Before embarking on further discussion of this topic, it is important to emphasise three points. Firstly, the goal of such education is not to teach or persuade students to adopt specific values, which would be wholly inappropriate and ethically dubious, but rather to assist students to develop the skills needed to identify and clarify their own personal and professional values.

Secondly, it is not possible or desirable that students

clarify their values in a static manner and then move on to another topic, with, as it were, their values remaining 'clarified'. Obviously, values are dynamic and may change over time with additional experiences. However, the intention is to assist students in understanding how values affect the positions they adopt in relation to certain issues, and to reflect in a systematic way on their own and other people's value positions in an ongoing manner.

Thirdly, emphasis should also be placed on the consequences of value positions for the individual, and for the effect that such positions may have on others.

What then is values clarification? The movement of values education was begun by Raths who was greatly influenced by Dewey, and in 1966, along with Harmin and Simon, wrote a seminal text, *Values and Teaching: Working with Values in the Classroom*. Raths defined values as the essential elements which show how one organises one's life. He then went on to specify the requirements necessary for a value to exist. These involve choosing, prizing and acting. Choosing involves freedom to select from a range of alternatives after a careful consideration of the consequences of each alternative. Prizing involves being proud of and happy with the choice and being prepared to affirm the choice publicly. Acting on values involves internalising or making the choice part of one's behaviour and repeating the choice in other situations.

Values clarification can, therefore, help in the analysis of feelings, beliefs and initial responses to situations and in the discovery of what is truly valued, by considering each of the points listed above. For example, throughout childhood, most people will have invariably been taught many 'values', and it may be that this acceptance of others' views is not consistent with the prevailing circumstances. This socialisation can lead to positions being adopted without any consideration being given to either the range of alternatives or the consequences of each of them. Frequently, it is only when individuals are called upon to affirm or justify their choices that they appreciate that not only do they not reflect their real beliefs or feelings, but also that they do not prize them. Simply asking students whether they are prepared to act on something that they say they value can increase their personal insight tremendously.

For teachers with little experience of values education, it may be expedient to incorporate prepared exercises into a programme of values clarification, rather than trying to devise one's own. Useful material can be found in texts by Tschudin (1992) and Hamilton and Kiefer (1986).

Specific content of courses

Having considered some of the precursors to ethics teaching, attention will now be given to the specific content which may feature in an ethics course.

There is currently much debate, especially in feminist literature, about the merit of approaches which emphasise specific principles such as autonomy, beneficence, non-maleficence, justice and rights, as opposed to those which emphasise an ethic of care. An alternative view is that it is only by introducing students to both of these approaches that they can be fully educated and be in a position to benefit from the writings and thoughts of others. It could be argued that to adopt one approach exclusively would leave the teacher open to the type of criticism that was alluded to earlier, namely that of indoctrination and manipulation.

It may be more effective if students are introduced to the major ethical theories such as utilitarianism, deontology and rights and the major ethical principles before being taught how these notions may be enhanced or modified by considerations of an approach based on care. Curtin (1983) illustrates this when she recounts a case involving a nurse who refuses to participate in the implantation of a cardiac pacemaker because the patient, an elderly, acutely confused woman, has refused consent. A second nurse, recognising that the refusal may be a direct result of the confusion, caused by a reduction in cardiac output, agrees to assist in the procedure and the woman is restored to health and the bosom of her family. This case shows clearly the limitations of adopting a principle approach (in this case the principle of autonomy) to the exclusion of other considerations, such as a concern for the actual well-being of the person, which an ethic of care emphasises.

Rather than principles, an ethic of care involves introducing concepts such as what it means to care, notions of commitment, obligation and responsiveness, the nature of caring relationships, self-sacrifice, dependence, empathy and involvement.

Following an introduction to the various approaches to ethics and the major theories and principles, it is important to consider the idea of professional norms and expectations. This can be done by exploring and comparing various nursing codes and contrasting these with the more general moral standards and norms within the wider society.

Next, students need to be given the opportunity to explore how the above content can be applied to the specific ethical problems that they are likely to face within their professional practice. It is useful if this can be done on both a societal and an individual level, as it is important that nurses appreciate that there is a need for them to be professionally involved in political debates in relation to health care and the formulation of health policy, as well as day-to-day issues in their own practice. For example, questions of resource allocation can be explored from a societal level by considering whether or not expensive techniques such as organ transplantation should be offered within a national health service. Resource implications can also be explored by taking a more local view, by involving

students in making decisions as to which patients should
have clean linen when there is only a limited supply, or
which clients should be given priority when staffing levels
are very low.

There is certainly no shortage of discussion or debate
topics and the following are examples of problems or issues
that might be included: the place of technology in care;
euthanasia; confidentiality; the value of conscience clauses;
whistleblowing; abortion; and resource allocation in
relation to different care groups, such as the mentally
handicapped or the elderly.

Finally, in addition to exploring concrete moral problems, students should be introduced to a critical scrutiny
of the social systems and economic structures in which, as
professional nurses, they will be required to operate.
Within this section, attention should be given to a consideration of the role and function of the profession of
nursing and the services which it offers to promote the
social good, the institutional settings in which such services
are delivered and the distribution of such services within
society. These topics are increasingly relevant in the light
of the current changes in the philosophy and organisation of the NHS and can serve to introduce students to
literature in political philosophy and social ethics. Having
decided on what will be taught, it is important to think
about how this content will be transmitted and learnt.

Choosing Appropriate Teaching and Learning Methods

The choice of teaching and learning methods is often a
result of a variety of factors such as class size, the availability
of accommodation, the nature of the content to be covered
and individual teacher and student preferences. Since the
advent of Project 2000, many nurses will be faced with

the challenge of teaching large intakes of students, often in excess of 100 in a single cohort, usually in inadequate accommodation and with a student–teacher ratio in excess of 15:1. In many colleges of nursing and midwifery, a large number of lectures have to be incorporated into the programme to enable a more favourable ratio for clinical teaching purposes.

As teachers, nurses will also have different personal skills and attributes which lend themselves more favourably to one teaching method rather than another, and, finally, students enter nursing from a wide range of backgrounds and vary in their abilities and interests. Despite these constraints, however, there are a variety of teaching methods which lend themselves particularly well to the topic of ethics.

Case studies

The use of case studies as a teaching strategy is extemely popular in many courses in applied ethics. This method allows students the opportunity to work through concrete dilemmas, so it can be extremely helpful in lending an aura of reality to what can be a highly abstract subject, especially if real problems or dilemmas from practice are used.

As well as illustrating specific points, case studies are probably most effective when used to highlight broader ethical principles and to develop consistent strategies for moral decision-making. For example, students can be given a blueprint by which to analyse each case, which requires that they proceed through the following stages: determining the facts that are known in the case; identifying the ethical problems, dilemmas or conflicts; considering the decisions that need to be made before any action can be taken; deciding on the criteria on which decisions should be based; determining who is best placed to make decisions; reflecting on alternative courses of action that may be appropriate; considering the likely outcomes of the various possible actions; and, finally, making and justifying an appropriate decision.

A further advantage of the case study approach is that the cases can be used in a variety of ways. Various aspects of the case can be role-played by students, after which a discussion that focuses on an analysis of the issues presented may follow. Videos and films can be shown supporting the case studies, and this can assist the students to identify common factors both in the case and in the supporting material. Multidisciplinary panels can be invited to debate the case with the student group. Depending on the case, the panel may consist of a senior nurse, a clinical nurse working in the specialty from which the case is drawn, a doctor, a chaplain, a philosopher, a lawyer or representatives of various pressure groups. This particular method has the added advantage of allowing students to hear varying perspectives and values in relation to the case and can also be valuable in developing skills in philosophical analysis and the presentation of arguments. Students themselves can present an analysis of individual cases in seminar sessions, where either an individual or small group is responsible for leading the discussion. Students frequently comment that they find this approach, although initially threatening, particularly effective as they are forced to focus on the issues and develop their own ideas and analytic skills.

Any readers wishing to explore the use of the case study as a method for ethics teaching should have no difficulty in finding suitable material. In addition to the increasing number of texts which adopt this approach (e.g. Melia, 1989; Rowson, 1990; Chadwick and Tadd, 1992) cases can also be drawn from the media, professional journals and incidents reported to the UKCC. However, probably the richest source of cases are nurses themselves; these cases can be collected in a number of ways from teaching colleagues, clinical staff or students. It is crucial that anonymity and confidentiality are maintained in this activity to protect all of the individuals concerned, and this requirement cannot be overemphasised.

The disadvantages of case studies

Having acclaimed the benefits of the case study method, there are however some potential disadvantages.

Firstly, students will often try to ascertain more facts about the case, claiming that if only they knew X, the solution would be clear. It is important, therefore, that the teacher insists that the facts remain as they are stated and also that students are helped to see that although it is vital that morally relevant facts are identified, having more facts does not necessarily make ethical dilemmas easier to resolve. Practising nurses have to grapple with hard cases in their day-to-day practice, and students need help and support to enable them to come to terms with this, rather than pretend that, with more knowledge, issues are always easier to deal with.

Secondly, students, and indeed qualified nurses, often fall into the trap of either trying to reduce ethical problems to clinical ones, as for example when discussing withholding an unfavourable diagnosis from a client, or focusing on the non-ethical aspects of particular cases, such as the benefits of one intervention rather than another. One of the major responsibilities of the teacher, therefore, is to ensure that during discussion of the case study, the debate remains focused on the ethical dimensions. The teacher also needs to be able to generalise from particular cases to show not only how similar issues may arise in different contexts, but also to emphasise morally relevant differences between cases. In this way, students' analytical and critical skills are heightened and their ability to recognise when issues are of an ethical nature is further developed.

Thirdly, within a classroom setting, it is all too easy to find a middle ground and remove the ethical dilemma, or to find other ways to avoid making a decision or finding a resolution. Thus, a useful ground rule to adopt when case studies are used is that, either as individuals or as small groups, a decision must always be taken in a case, along with a justification as to why it was chosen. This also emphasises to students that, in practice, prevarication is rarely an option that is available.

The final point to be aware of in relation to the use of case studies is that there can be an initial tendency to use very dramatic cases, which clearly illustrate the issues involved. This can be counterproductive in that the emotional reaction can be so strong that students find it difficult to undertake a calm analysis of the issues. Also, the exclusive use of sensational material can foster in students the idea that ethics has no part to play in everyday practice. By incorporating examples of cases from the day-to-day experience of clinical nurses, this is avoided, and students are helped to see the central role that ethics plays in everyday professional practice.

Other teaching methods

The lecture remains one of the most effective methods of giving essential information to large numbers of students, although its major disadvantage is that opportunities for class discussion are necessarily restricted, although not totally negated. One very useful book, packed full of ideas for increasing student involvement and activities which are particularly appropriate in ethics sessions, is *53 Interesting Things To Do in Your Lectures* (Gibb, Habeshaw and Habeshaw, 1988).

Where the lecture plays a central role is in the presentation of major concepts and in introducing students to the literature. Introduction to the serious literature is even more crucial if case studies are to be used extensively, as an appropriate balance needs to be found between cases and theoretical material.

Another very effective teaching method is the debate, whereby students have the opportunity to support and oppose motions which can be developed by the teacher or by the students themselves. Adequate preparation time must be given to the students, and initially it is desirable that the proceedings be chaired by the teacher, unless the students are experienced in formal debating. It can also be beneficial for students to have to justify a position with which they do not agree, as this encourages them to consider others' viewpoints and sharpens their analytical and presentational skills.

Workshops can be used to stimulate critical thinking by focusing on multidimensional problems that help students to incorporate learning from other subject areas, along with considerations of ethics. For example, problems which enable students to explore aspects of quality, audit, skill mix, health promotion and changes in the NHS all serve to demonstrate the pervasive nature of ethics in our personal and professional lives and help to highlight the importance of the topic to them not only as practising nurses, but also as individual moral agents.

As students become more familiar with the topic and less embarrassed at putting forward their views, an ethics awareness group can be formed as an extracurricular activity for those with a particular interest in this area.

Role modelling

The term role model is not meant to suggest that teachers should set themselves up as a paragon of virtue. However, it is essential to recognise that students are unlikely to accept statements about the centrality of ethics to nursing if they are not treated with respect and fairness by the individual staff members and within the institutional policies and educational frameworks. It is, therefore, worth considering the opportunities that are provided within the college to promote student empowerment and rights within the curricular processes. For instance, are students represented on evaluation and monitoring committees? Are mechanisms available for students to raise issues and concerns? The institutional philosophy should ensure that respect and consideration, the provision of encouragement and support, the instillation of feelings of self-worth, and the setting of clear limits and expectations underlie all activities, as these are as important as the explicit teaching which takes place.

Ensuring that students experience care within their professional education is a powerful way in which to teach the relevance of an ethic of care. Imagine the effect on a group of students who after sitting through a session on confidentiality overhear a teacher ridiculing one of their assignments, or who are taught about respect for persons by a teacher who is repeatedly late for class or who never gives back marked assignments. Noddings (1984) emphasises caring as the essential way of being to which every other educational aim must be subservient, when she states that:

> The primary aim of every educational institution and of
> every educational effort must be the maintenance and
> enhancement of caring. . . It functions as end, means
> and criterion for judging suggested means. It establishes
> the climate, a first approximation to the range of acceptable
> practices, and a lens through which all practices and
> possible practices are examined.

Her sentiments are particularly significant for nurse education, and, perhaps, when teaching ethics, the old adage that actions speak louder than words really does apply.

When To Teach Ethics

There is probably no single answer to the question of when is the best time to introduce an ethics component into the nursing curriculum, as this will largely depend upon how it is organised. What is possibly more important than when is that students should have the opportunity to undertake a systematic study of ethics at some point in their programme. Gallagher and Boyd (1991) discovered that in 80 per cent of pre-registration courses studied, ethics teaching was integrated with other subjects and mainly appeared to be informal in nature, relying heavily on students and teachers raising issues at appropriate times. Seventy-four per cent of the centres surveyed offered four hours or less, and only two centres devoted more than 10 hours to the teaching of ethics.

The danger of ethics being taught as a separate subject is that it will become compartmentalised. It is an unfortunate fact that students tend to view the subjects within the timetable as discrete areas of learning. This results in the erroneous reasoning that just as psychology is only discussed in psychology lectures, so nursing ethics can only be addressed in ethics lectures.

However, the difficulty with relying solely on an integrated approach to ethics teaching is that students are unlikely to gain a thorough understanding of the nature and language of ethics, nor will they be able to acquire an understanding of the relationship between ethical theories and principles and actual moral problems and dilemmas. Such an approach assumes that everyone is competent to teach ethics and, at the same time, denies that ethics constitutes a form of knowledge in its own right. Without the thorough understanding which some discrete teaching can offer, students will be less likely to feel comfortable or confident about entering into ethical debates, let alone embarking on informed and effective ethical decision-making.

It is doubtful whether there is one correct answer on whether ethics ought to be taught as a separate subject or integrated into other teaching. Probably the best outcomes are achieved by incorporating aspects of both approaches. Students entering the common foundation programme could, for example, undertake a brief introductory unit on philosophy and philosophical method, utilising lectures, student-led seminars and small group tutorials. In the author's institution, this accounts for approximately 18 hours of teaching time, being equally divided between formal and informal sessions. The early introduction of philosophy enables students to utilise newly-acquired skills in other subject areas and, in particular, prepares them to formulate and raise pertinent questions. The philosophy unit is followed by a unit concerning ethical aspects of health care. This also incorporates lecture and small group teaching and covers some 30 hours of teaching time. One third of this is spent in lectures, with the remainder divided between seminars, workshops and debates, which all facilitate student involvement, interaction and the development of reasoning.

Within two of the branch programmes, separate units on ethical aspects in relation to the specific care group are then undertaken, while in the two remaining branches, ethical issues arising in the particular specialty are explored in an integrated manner throughout the branch programme. A further common unit explores the notion of professional accountability in more depth across each of the four branches.

In time, it may prove to be the case that those who have undertaken separate units within the branch programmes will be less able to appreciate the pervasive nature of ethics, seeing it as a topic to be explored in isolation. In those branches where no specific unit has been identified, the integration of ethics content may well not occur because teaching time is at a premium. In addition, teachers without special interest or competence may find it difficult or particularly challenging to be expected to discuss ethical aspects of care at any great depth, especially with students who may be better prepared than they are to explore the issues. It will be interesting to evaluate at the end of all the branch programmes which method has best succeeded in preparing students to face ethical dilemmas encountered in their practice.

Another frequent debate is whether ethics teaching should occur earlier or later in a course. Again, there are advantages and disadvantages to be considered. If ethics is taught at the beginning of a course, it is unlikely that students will have the necessary clinical experience, or a sufficient understanding of the nature of their chosen profession and its current problems, to be able fully to debate issues. On the other hand, teaching ethics early in the programme not only signifies the importance placed on ethics, but also enables and encourages students to identify the ethical aspects of their practice as soon as they enter the clinical areas. Thinking about potential moral problems before being faced with them is one way of preparing students to deal with moral distress before it is encountered. If only one place for teaching can be identified within the course, it is probably better that ethics is introduced earlier rather than later.

Who Should Teach Ethics?

This question probably arises more frequently in nurse education than it does in any other educational setting.

Within readers' own institutions, colleagues can no doubt be found debating whether psychology or sociology should be taught by purists in the discipline or by nurses who, having studied the subject at an advanced level, are better able to apply the specific knowledge of the discipline to nursing. The debate follows exactly the same line of argument when it is applied to the teaching of ethics.

As nursing increasingly moves into higher education, these debates will no doubt increase, as, in the past, nurse teachers have invariably found themselves teaching a whole range of subjects, rather than being allowed the luxury of specialisation. Although many colleagues claim that teaching from such a broad base has been one of the strengths of the nurse teacher, others argue that it has led to students of nursing knowing a little about many subjects, none of them in depth. Thus, to some extent the process of forging closer links with colleagues in higher education, and the enforced specialisation and change in teaching emphasis that this has involved, have induced feelings of uncertainty and threat which can be increased when teachers have to teach subjects for which they have had little preparation.

Despite interest and eagerness being important requisites for every teacher, they do not together constitute sufficient qualification for the teaching of ethics or, for that matter, psychology, sociology, physiology or law. This does not mean that to teach ethics satisfactorily, one requires only an academic training in philosophy or ethics. Such a background would not provide the necessary appreciation and understanding of the practical moral problems faced by nurses. Similarly, a nurse teacher without any formal introduction to philosophy or ethical theory is unlikely to be sufficiently familiar with the literature or to have grasped the language, concepts and methods of analysis necessary for teaching the subject effectively.

One approach that can be particularly effective,

especially when the nurse teacher lacks specialist prep-aration, and providing that adequate resources can be allo-cated, is to use 'team teaching' or joint sessions, involving both a nurse and a philosopher. This can also be very successful in teaching philosophy, as technical aspects can be thoroughly explained by the philosopher and the practi-cal application can be emphasised by the nurse. In this way, technical correctness is not sacrificed to application in nursing, and the pragmatic value of philosophy or ethics is not lost because sessions become too abstract.

For those teachers who wish to develop expertise in ethics, a number of postgraduate courses are available in health care and other branches of applied ethics, most of which are offered in the major centres throughout the UK on a part-time basis. With the advent of the Centre for Applied Ethics in Cardiff, along with others through-out the UK, interest by the National Boards for Nursing, Midwifery and Health Visiting in developing post-regis-tration courses is growing; these can also provide suitable introductory courses for teachers interested in the topic area.

In addition to formal courses, organisations such as the Society of Applied Philosophy, the International Associ-ation of Bioethics and the Royal College of Nursing offer workshops, conferences, international networks and forums for nurses, which provide ideal starting points to gain information and make contact with others who have similar interests.

Assessment in Ethics

Despite the claim by many teachers involved in nurse education that ethics is an important component of the curriculum, relatively few colleges require any formal assessment of competence in ethics (Gallagher and Boyd,

1991). The consequences of this are important as students frequently determine the relative importance of subjects according to whether or not they are assessed. The lack of any formal assessment in ethics may, therefore, give implicit messages about the professional value placed on this aspect of nursing practice, and this factor alone provides a very powerful reason why ethics, like other topics, should be the subject of both formal and informal assessment.

An obvious mode of assessment is that of essay or assignment writing, in which the abilities to identify ethical issues, to apply ethical theory to practical concerns, to mount logical and coherent arguments and to demonstrate an understanding of the literature can all be readily scrutinised. This method can not only be used to provide the students with informal feedback on their performance but also constitutes an acceptable means of formal assessment.

There are, however, additional methods which should not be overlooked. One of these, which has been used very successfully, is self-assessment. This can be used both in relation to theoretical learning — where students assess what they have learned from a single session — and also as part of a continuing assessment scheme. In the latter application, students identify when they have achieved specific targets and provide their mentors or preceptors with evidence to substantiate their claims. This evidence can be drawn from written accounts of practice in course journals or from student learning profiles. The use of self-evaluation has the additional bonus of encouraging systematic reflection on performance and learning, which is an essential skill if nurses are to continue to flourish and develop professionally after registration.

Theoretical assessment is, however, only part of the equation. In nursing, as in many other professions, it is important that nurses approach their practice in an ethical manner. Clinical assessment, therefore, requires attention, more especially because in practice the distinction between teaching, learning and assessment becomes less clear cut. The introduction of supernumerary status with Project 2000 has meant that it is somewhat easier for nurse teachers to manage the students' clinical learning, depending on how the curriculum is organised. In many colleges, clinical experience commences with regular but brief exposures to practice, where the emphasis is on learning clinical skills, prior to longer placements in patient areas, in which students have the opportunity to practise and consolidate their learning.

From the outset, the ethical dimensions of patient care should be highlighted and students encouraged to discuss these aspects with both their supervisors and clinical staff, in much the same way that the technical, psychological and physical elements of care are introduced and discussed. As students gain in their confidence and clinical competence, it requires only a slight shift in emphasis to move from discussion with the students to questioning and direct assessment. Such assessment can focus on the identification of ethical issues, the possible actions that are open to the health care team and which actions have been chosen, why and by whom. In this way, the importance of this vital aspect of care is emphasised rather than merely being an interesting theoretical activity. The ethical aspect of care thus becomes a live issue and part of the day-to-day life of the nurse, especially when documentation of such activity is required as part of the formal clinical assessment.

One difficulty of introducing direct questioning on ethics into the process of clinical assessment is the lack of knowledge and experience of many teachers and practitioners. To some extent, this can be overcome by adequate preparation prior to the students' clinical visits. Teachers responsible for teaching the theoretical content can undertake ethics rounds (Mahon and Everson, 1979), which involve the presentation and discussion of current patient case studies in those clinical areas that are to be used by students. These can be shared by teachers and clinical staff, and gradually the responsibility for presentation and discussion can be shouldered by the participants. The sessions should last no longer than an hour and thus not pose a major strain on resources. They have the added advantage of providing a valuable means of continuing education by drawing the attention of qualified staff to issues which, in the hurly-burly of daily routine, may go unnoticed.

The Implications of Ethics Teaching

The implications of introducing formal ethics education into the curriculum fall into two categories — those which mainly affect the individuals concerned and those which mainly affect the institution — although it needs to be emphasised that this categorisation is not entirely discrete.

Teachers have to consider how they will deal with students who come to see them as opponents in the classroom if sessions are not to become battles of the wills or, alternatively, monologues by the teacher. Because of the nature of ethics, the teacher is often in the position of highlighting deficiencies in the arguments that students put forward. This is, in fact, one way in which students learn to improve their skills. This may, however, have negative results if students come to believe that because of their training, teachers can make any view look good or bad, leading to the mistaken idea that ethics is simply a matter of technical expertise and opinion, and, therefore, that all views are equally correct. Teachers should be prepared to show that not all moral views are equally correct and also that there is no contradiction involved when one claims that all views have a right to be heard. One way of avoiding this is to evade presenting single solutions to problems but instead to show a range of possible solutions and the deficiencies which exist within each of them. This should also be reinforced in sessions in which the class is involved in the communal effort of comparing or considering theories, rather than acting as individuals.

One of the main implications of ethics teaching has already been discussed, namely that during their educational preparation, nursing students need to be treated fairly and with respect by both the teaching staff and the institutional policies. Possibly more than any other staff member, the person responsible for teaching ethics will be called upon to justify institutional rules, because ethics is about justification. For instance, rules about handing in and marking of assignments, attendance and student classroom contribution will no doubt be aired, and teachers need to consider how they will answer or handle criticisms in a constructive manner if, or rather when, they arise.

An even greater difficulty for the teacher to contend with is when students ask why they should be moral, or worse, how they can be moral, bearing in mind the institutional constraints which the majority of professionals have to face. One can pick up almost any recent edition of a popular nursing journal and read letters or news items in relation to the fate of whistleblowers or those wishing to express concern about poor standards. In many examples, the complainant becomes the victim, not only antagonising employers, but also being seen as disloyal by colleagues, a number of whom may themselves be feeling guilty because they were prepared to turn a blind eye to indifferent care practices, out of either expediency or ignorance. In the past, nurses who have summoned up the courage to complain about poor standards of care have been labelled as trouble makers by senior managers and thus have hardly promoted their chances of career development. Not only does the individual suffer, but also family members can pay a high price, as the nurse may well take home the stresses and strains that she or he is experiencing.

Teachers need to recognise that this is where the interface between individual and institutional implications may overlap, as one potential result of incorporating ethics teaching may well be an increased incidence in the reporting of inadequate standards of care.

Supporting the nurses

As the fundamental aim of ethics teaching is to promote the patient's interests, it would be futile, if not actually immoral, to invest time and expensive resources in preparing nursing students and qualified practitioners, if they were then to remain silent when improvements in care practices were found to be necessary. Indeed, the UKCC has recently issued guidance to purchasers and providers of health services in relation to recognition of the Code of Professional Conduct in the employment contracts of nurses, support for staff enabling them to satisfy the requirements of the Code, and agreements to honour the individual nurse's right to freedom of speech (UKCC 1992b). Students need, therefore, to be adequately prepared to make complaints, and, as they are particularly vulnerable, it would be equally immoral if, having raised concerns, students were left to shoulder the responsibility without adequate support. Thus, teachers may need to be prepared to act as advocates, ensuring that student complaints are taken seriously.

With regard to institutional implications, a consequence of the rationalisation of schools of nursing into large colleges spanning a number of health districts, and the changes in the purchaser–provider relationships within health authorities, has been that the old reference points between service and education have been lost. It is even more important, therefore, that these factors are aired with senior staff in clinical placements and that, where necessary, nurse managers formulate procedures to deal with complaints in a constructive and open manner.

Support mechanisms should also be established for staff who discover that standards of care have fallen below the minimal requirements. One method of both supporting and educating staff is by broadening the remit of established ethical committees. Rather than merely reviewing research protocols, which has been the traditional focus of such groups, these committees might usefully discuss issues raised by staff and, where appropriate, distribute guidance.

Other important institutional considerations that should not be overlooked include the need for continuing education. If the teaching of ethics is to be more than a paper exercise, it is essential that clinical staff are not only knowledgeable about ethical theory, but must also be prepared to practise in an ethical manner. As key people in the education of students, qualified nurses are powerful role models for junior staff. It would be unfair and unreasonable to expect practitioners to acquire the necessary knowledge and insights overnight, without additional help and support. Therefore, resources and opportunities that emphasise this aspect of nursing care need to be provided to support programmes of continuing education. Indeed, it could be argued that this is a priority, as ethical care must be an essential component of quality care. If considerations of quality are so important as to be regarded as major requirements of service contracts, it is imperative that senior managers realise that the professional development of nurses needs to be viewed as an investment rather than as a financial burden.

A further implication concerns the monitoring of the learning environment. The curriculum embraces more than that which is taught within the classroom; it also comprises the experiences which the student undertakes, so the clinical areas must reflect the stated educational outcomes. One method of determining the suitability of the various experiences is that of educational audit, and just as a clinical area might be deemed unsuitable were resources for the delivery of physical care inadequate, it might be equally unsuitable were the ethical climate found to be lacking. For example, it is of little value that the Code of Professional Conduct is pinned on the ward notice board if, on being questioned, qualified staff have no idea of what it entails. It is essential, therefore, that the educational audit includes a section covering the 'ethical environment' of care. However, audits usually occur only once per year, while staffing and other changes are taking place almost continually. One of the most important roles of the nurse teacher within the clinical area is, therefore, the continued monitoring of the learning milieu. Only when all of these implications have been fully addressed can the full potential teaching of ethics be achieved.

Conclusion

Although in the past the professional education of nurses in the humanities generally, and in ethics in particular, has been neglected, there are signs that, at last, this is changing. The inclusion of ethics in the nursing curriculum should mean that in future not only will nurses be better prepared to make the moral judgements that are required of them every day of their working lives, but also that they will be able to participate as equal partners in making decisions about patient care. All too often, nurses have failed to express their professional point of view, both to senior nurses and to other members of the care team. To some extent, this has been due to their inability to formulate and express rational arguments, relying instead on emotional and intuitive responses, which can be all too readily dimissed as illogical.

The challenges and constraints facing the health service today mean that, more than ever, nurses need to assert their importance in providing a humane and caring environment in which the needs of patients and clients can be safely met. An understanding of ethics can help to create a body of knowledge about care, which, in turn, can free nurses from their dependence on medicine's cure-based approach to health care. This is where the nurse's true professionalism lies and, as such, it provides a route to nursing's autonomy, which in the words of Downey and Kelly (1978), 'is the ability to make choices on controversial issues of value . . . as a result of one's own thinking. It is in essence moral autonomy'.

References

Brown J M, Kitson A L and McKnight T J (1992) *Challenges in Caring*. London: Chapman and Hall.

Chadwick R and Tadd W (1992) *Ethics in Nursing Practice: a Case-study Approach*. London: Macmillan.

Curtin L L (1983) The nurse as advocate: a cantankerous critique. *Nursing Management*, 14: pp. 9–10.

Dewey J (1910) *How We Think*. Lexington, Mass: Heath.

Downey M and Kelly A V (1978) *Moral Education, Theory and Practice*. New York: Harper and Row.

Gallagher U and Boyd K M (1991) *Teaching and Learning Nursing Ethics*. London: Scutari Press.

Gibb G, Habeshaw S and Habeshaw T (1988) *53 Interesting Things To Do in Your Lectures* (3rd edn.). Bristol: Technical and Educational Services Ltd.

Hamilton J M and Kiefer M E (1986) *Survival Skills for the New Nurse*. Philadelphia: J B Lippincott.

Hunt G (1991) *Moral Responsibility and the Nurse*. Unpublished conference paper. London: National Centre for Nursing and Midwifery Ethics.

Mahon K and Everson S (1979) Moral outrage — nurses right

or responsibility: ethical rounds for nurses. *Journal of Continuing Education in Nursing*, 10: pp. 4–7.

Melia K M (1989) *Everyday Nursing Ethics*. Basingstoke: Macmillan.

Murdoch I (1970) *The Sovereignty of Good*. London: Routledge and Kegan Paul.

Noddings N (1984) *Caring: a Feminine Approach to Ethics and Moral Education*. Berkeley, California: University of California Press.

Raths L E, Harmin M and Simon S B (1966) *Values and Teaching: Working with Values in the Classroom*. Columbus, Ohio: Merrill.

Rowson R H (1990) *An Introduction to Ethics for Nurses*. London: Scutari Press.

Seedhouse D (1988) *Ethics: the Heart of Health Care*. Chichester: John Wiley and Sons.

Statutory Instruments (1989) no. 1456. *Nurses, Midwives and Health Visitors (Registered Fever Nurses) Amendment Rules* 1989, Rule 18A.

Strawson P (1982) Freedom and resentment. In G Warson (ed.) *Free Will*. Oxford: Oxford University Press.

Taylor P (1975) *Principles of Ethics: an Introduction*. Belmont, California: Wadsworth.

Tschudin V (1992) *Values: a Primer for Nurses (Workbook)*. London: Baillière Tindall.

UKCC (1983) *Code of Professional Conduct for the Nurse, Midwife and Health Visitor* (1st edn.). London: UKCC.

UKCC (1984) *Code of Professional Conduct for the Nurse, Midwife and Health Visitor* (2nd edn.). London: UKCC.

UKCC (1989) *Exercising Accountability.* London: UKCC.

UKCC (1992a) *Code of Professional Conduct* (3rd edn.). London: UKCC.

UKCC (1992b) *Registrar's Letter and Annexe 37/1992: Standards for Incorporation into Contracts for Hospital and Community Health Care Services*. London: UKCC.

Further Reading

Baker E (1973) On teaching ethics to nurses. *Nursing Times*, May 24: pp. 683–4.

Clay M and Povey R (1983) Moral reasoning and the student nurse. *Journal of Advanced Nursing*, 8 (4): pp. 297–302.

Jarrett J L (1991) *The Teaching of Values: Caring and Appreciation.* London: Routledge.

Johnson M (1983) Ethics in nurse education — a comment. *Nurse Education Today*, 3 (3): pp. 58–9.

Kay B (1991) 'I nurse therefore. . .', *Nursing Standard*, 5 (20): pp. 54–5.

Langford M J (1990) The Moot Court in teaching bioethics. *Nurse Education Today*, 10 (1): pp. 24–30.

Meyers C (1986) *Teaching Students To Think Critically.* San Francisco: Jossey-Bass.

Tadd W and Chadwick R (1989) Philosophical analysis and its value to the nurse teacher. *Nurse Education Today*, 9 (3): pp. 155–60.

CHAPTER 2

Nursing Research

Diane Marks-Maran

Nursing is more and more becoming a research-based profession. But what sort of research is it, and how is it done?

A simple piece of research has given the author the basis to argue for looking at research in a different way. This chapter leads the reader to new vistas of nursing, caring and research. Readers, including those not engaged (or perhaps not even interested) in research, will find this chapter clear, unexpected, challenging and thought-provoking.

It is well documented in the nursing literature (Rumbold, 1986; Johnstone, 1989; Tschudin, 1992; Tschudin and Marks–Maran, 1993) that within all spheres of nursing practice, ethical issues, questions and dilemmas arise. Nurses' ability to cope with ethical dilemmas relating to practice depends on their having a good understanding of their own values and feelings as well as a certain amount of knowledge of ethics and ethical principles and their application to real situations at work.

Research, too, raises a number of ethical issues, problems and potential dilemmas. As for nursing practice, coping with ethical issues in research requires nurses to examine their values and feelings as well as to apply knowledge of ethics and ethical principles to research-related ethical situations.

This chapter will explore five areas concerning ethics and nursing research:

- an overview of the relationship between ethical principles and research;

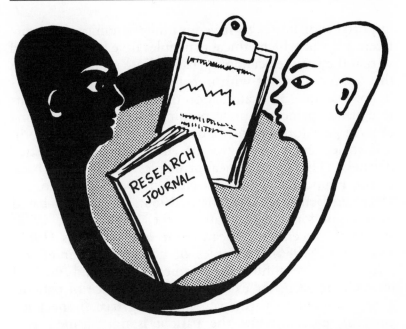

- ethical issues for the nurse who is carrying out research;
- ethical issues for those in positions of authority where nursing research is undertaken;
- ethical issues related to nurses' involvement in other people's research;
- the ethical issues of using or not using research findings.

An Overview of the Relationship Between Ethical Principles and Nursing Research

Two key points are important to consider here. Firstly, the ethical principles applied to nursing research are the same principles that are applied to nursing practice. Secondly, throughout history the literature describes different taxonomies for identifying ethical principles. It is, therefore, important for nurses to have an understanding of the different ways in which ethical principles have been identified so that they can select appropriately those ethical principles that seem congruent with nursing practice and research.

For example, an examination of the literature highlights four ethical principles underpinning medical ethics: autonomy/respect for persons; beneficence (duty to do good); non-maleficence (duty to do no harm); and justice (fairness). These four ethical principles can be traced back to the Hippocratic Oath (as cited in Davis and Aroskar, 1983 and Benjamin and Curtis, 1986), to the duty-based theory put forward by Kant in the 1700s (Kant, 1972) and, more recently, to Beauchamp and Childress (1983) and Gillon (1986). Examples of how these four ethical principles have influenced medical ethics and medical research are seen, for example, in the practice of patients giving consent to participate in a drug trial (respect for persons), ensuring that the patient is not harmed as a result of participating in any research (non-maleficence), demonstrating that participation in the research is in the best interests of the patient (beneficence), and using random sampling and blind/double blind techniques to select patients and control bias in drug trials (justice/fairness). Whether it is appropriate to use these same ethical principles and to apply these principles to *nursing* research remains to be seen. What is interesting to note is that ethics committees, in considering medical research trials, use the beneficence *v* non-maleficence balance in making their decisions. Questions can be asked as to whether these same ethical criteria are appropriate to ethical scrutiny of nursing research. This will be examined later in this chapter.

There has been an attempt in recent years to assume that the above four ethical principles also underpin nursing ethics (Thompson, Melia and Boyd, 1983; Melia, 1989), the assumption being that medical ethics and nursing ethics are the same. However, Johnstone (1989) makes the point that:

> although the facts and concerns of these two disciplines overlap in many areas, they are ideologically separate in their endeavours, and it would be incorrect to treat them as being synonymous.

Johnstone continues this argument by pointing out that bioethics, biomedical ethics and medical ethics are not one and the same thing, a view first put forward by Veatch (1985). At best, medical ethics is a subsection of bioethics, just as nursing is a separate subsection of bioethics (Johnstone, 1987). It is this ideological separateness of nursing and medicine that perhaps begins to indicate that the ethical principles underpinning medicine and medical ethics are, indeed, different from the ethical principles underpinning nursing and nursing research.

So to what alternative taxonomies of ethical principles, which may be more ideologically congruent with nursing and nursing research, might nurses turn?

One of the simplest ideological differentiations between nursing and medicine that has been proposed is the notion that medicine is primarily about 'cure', while nursing is about 'care'. Roach (1987) calls this care/cure distinction a false dichotomy because caring is not unique to any particular profession. However, in a recent unpublished survey (not referenced), the author asked groups of nurses to write down words which described what nursing is. One hundred per cent of the nurses (from a total of 41) cited the word 'care' or 'caring' in their first two choices of words. Groups of doctors were asked to write down words that described for them what medical practice was. Fewer than 1 per cent of respondents (from a total of 29) cited the words 'care' or 'caring' in their lists. The author does not conclude that doctors do not care; the inference, however, is that when asked, the majority of doctors do not view their primary role as 'caring'. So if there is an argument for suggesting that cure is different from care and that nursing is about 'caring', it could follow that medical (curing) ethics is indeed different from nursing (caring) ethics.

As an alternative to the four duty-based ethical principles described earlier in this chapter, Thiroux (1980) identifies a different taxonomy of five ethical principles:

- The value of life (human beings should revere life and accept death).
- Goodness or rightness (promoting good over bad, causing no badness, preventing badness).
- Justice or fairness (equal distribution of goodness and badness across all people).
- Truth-telling or honesty.
- Individual freedom (freedom of individuals to choose their own ways of being moral within the framework of the other four principles).

If one were to begin to apply Thiroux's ethical principles to nursing research and the nurse's role in research, these are some of the questions that nurses may ask in order to examine the ethics of their nursing practice or nursing research:

- Does this research, or my participation in the research, promote goodness, cause harm or prevent harm from happening?
- Does this research, or my participation in the research, ensure that the time or activities involved in the research do not take me away from 'doing good' for this or any other patient?
- To what extent have I been completely honest with the patient about the research?
- To what extent do I enable patients to make their

own moral choices about participating in the research?

Another alternative approach to identifying ethical principles, which may be more suitable to nursing and nursing research (as suggested above), is based on the concept of caring. Tschudin (1992) cites Roach (1987) when making the point that the most ethical response a nurse can give in any situation is that which is the most caring response. 'Caring', however, as a concept, can be quite elusive. Roach identified five characteristics of caring. These are:

- compassion;
- competence;
- confidence;
- conscience;
- commitment.

Although Roach makes no claims that the above five characteristics of caring are ethical principles, they can be used as an alternative way of examining what constitutes ethical behaviour in nursing and nursing research.

Compassion

Nouwen (1982) writes:

Compassion requires us to be weak with the weak [and] vulnerable with the vulnerable.

Compassion is not just about kindness; it is about sharing hurt and pain and being fully immersed in the condition of being human. In a research context, it is about not losing sight of people's feelings, weaknesses or vulnerability in the quest for new knowledge. It is also about recognising that conflict can arise when a nurse in the role of researcher experiences conflict with her or his role as carer. This problem will be further addressed later in this chapter.

Competence

Competence can be described as the state of having the experience, skill, judgement and wisdom to respond appropriately. Roach (1987) calls for competence with a caring face, a notion which applies as much to the research role of the nurse as the care-giving role. As an ethical concept, competence is about two things: being aware of the level of competence required for a certain nursing activity (e.g. research) and distinguishing between using knowledge, skill, experience and wisdom for caring rather than for power over others. These apply both to the practice of nursing and to nursing research.

Confidence

Confidence is described by Roach (1987) as the quality which fosters trusting relationships. The ethical principle underpinning this is that of fidelity (trust). Patients entrust themselves to the care of nurses, whether those nurses are in the role of care-giver or researcher. This sense of trust is based on their belief that nurses will act in such a way as to safeguard patients' interests. This is known in ethical terms as a fiduciary relationship and is echoed by the UKCC (1992), which states that the nurse must:

> Act always in such a manner as to promote and safeguard the interests and well-being of patients and clients.

Confidence, then, is the security patients have in knowing that the principle of fidelity will be upheld within this fiduciary relationship.

Confidence is also linked to honesty or truth-telling as an ethical principle. A trusting (fiduciary) relationship rests upon the degree of honesty that each party in the relationship is perceived to exhibit. Bok (1978) observes that there is a lack of emphasis on truth-telling in medical codes of practice. If ethical nursing practice and research within the notion of *confidence* is to be taken seriously, truth-telling needs to be a serious aspect of nursing and research practice.

Conscience

Tschudin (1992) describes conscience as a state of moral awareness. Roach (1987) defines it as 'The caring person attuned to the moral nature of things'. Conscience is that part of us which is the embodiment of our values and our sense of right and wrong and good or bad. Conscience, according to Roach, is the medium through which morality is personalised. Conscience is also a state of loyalty to one's sense of right and wrong. At best, it prompts an individual to choose a morally right response over other options; at the very least, it tells us quite strongly when, due to other pressures, we have chosen to respond in a way that, deep down, is contrary to that which we believe to be morally right.

The notion of moral rightness requires extensive discussion to comprehend it fully — more than is possible in this chapter. Johnstone (1989) attempts to distinguish between what is 'right' from a moral perspective and from other perspectives. She differentiates moral rightness from that which may be legally right, managerially right or 'right' in terms of professional etiquette. She also distinguishes between what is morally right and what the majority say is right, as well as distinguishing between what is morally right and what is a 'gut response'. Johnstone makes these varying distinctions in order to encourage nurses to differentiate between following moral convictions and responding to other rules or pressures. Johnstone makes the point that:

> If nurses fail to distinguish ethics from these, they risk not only failing to prevent moral errors and harms from

occurring in health care domains, but may actually cause them to occur.

It is conscience that enables individuals to distinguish between moral rightness and other pressures and rules.

Commitment

Tschudin (1992) defines commitment as 'that certain "stickability" which gets a person involved with another person or task. . .'. Commitment is more than just a willingness to do something; it is a choice which is so strong that the decision is synonymous with what an individual really wants to do. In moral terms, commitment is a desire to act in a caring way, which is based on firmly valuing that action and really wanting to behave in that way. Mayeroff (1971) refers to this type of commitment as 'devotion'. If commitment to care is a strong value, the nurse researcher can transfer this caring commitment to her or his research work and thus bring caring commitment into research activity as well as practice.

These 'Five C's' of caring (compassion, competence, confidence, conscience and commitment) were not intended by Roach (1987) to be seen as ethical principles. However, they do offer an alternative perspective to making moral choices as a nurse practitioner or as a nurse involved in research.

Tschudin (1992) describes caring as the basis for nursing ethics. This can be extended to include ethics in nursing research. A value system is part of who a person is, and, as such, to embrace a caring ethic as a nurse practitioner is to embrace the same ethic when involved with research.

Unlike Roach, Johnstone says categorically that care is an ethical principle and that, when placed in context, it offers Western moral philosophy a new and vital direction of enquiry (Johnstone, 1989). Johnstone was writing about feminist moral theory as an alternative to Western theory, and went on to suggest that although principles such as care, compassion, empathy, friendship and sympathy have been identified as being valid components of an alternative moral theory, they do not as yet form a substantive ethical theory.

The object of such alternative approaches to ethics is to move towards approaches that take into account the reality of the circumstances of life — a kind of 'grounded ethical theory'. Johnstone also points out that such approaches to ethical theory recognise the strengths of both masculine and feminine moral perceptions (Kohlberg, 1981; Gilligan, 1987). The author suggests that alternative ethical theories related to health care need also to take into account the strengths of both medical (masculine) and nursing (feminine) moral perceptions.

Historically, the major ethical traditions in medical ethics and medical research ethics have arisen out of a masculine, isolationist viewpoint. Deontologists (e.g. Kant) might ask 'What ought I to do for my research to be ethically correct?', while utilitarians might ask 'What is the aim of my research?'. These approaches form the basis for historical and current approaches to medical ethics.

An alternative approach based on the principles of caring (Roach, 1987; Johnstone, 1989) is to ask the question 'What is the most caring response to an ethical issue in my involvement with this research?'. Niebuhr (1963) argued for just such an approach, which he calls 'response ethics' and which aims to show that the most ethical response in any situation is the one which leads to a sense of community.

The kinds of ethical question related to involvement in research which nurses might ask, using the principles of caring, are:

- does my participation in this research impinge on the caring and compassion I can offer my patient? ;
- how can I be a caring researcher? ;
- does my participation in this research undermine the trust my patient puts in me? ;
- how can I resolve the conflict between my caring commitment to my patient and my desire to increase my knowledge of caring through research? ;
- what does my conscience tell me is the morally right approach to this research?

This first section of this chapter has attempted to offer an overview of traditional approaches to medical and nursing ethics and some alternative approaches. The remaining sections will specifically examine four aspects of ethics related to nursing research: nurses undertaking research; nurses in positions of authority in research settings; involvement of nurses in other people's research; and using (or not using) research findings in nursing practice.

Nurses Undertaking Research

The RCN guidelines for nursing research (RCN, 1993) identify three areas of consideration for nurses who are undertaking research. These are:

- the personal and professional integrity of the researcher;
- responsibility of nurse researchers to their subjects;
- relationships with sponsors, employers and colleagues.

The personal and professional integrity of the researcher

The Concise Oxford Dictionary (1976) defines integrity as:

wholeness; entirety; soundness; uprightness; honesty.

It is the last two words of this definition — 'uprightness; honesty' — which are of relevance to an exploration of the integrity of the nurse carrying out research. Flaherty (1982) defines integrity as 'doing what one believes to be right, regardless of the cost'.

As a definition, integrity is closely related to conscience, since integrity within one's research activities is similar to Tschudin's (1992) 'conscience as a state of moral awareness' and Roach's (1987) definition of conscience as 'the caring person attuned to the moral nature of things'. Integrity is, therefore, more than what a person does; it is also about how much insight a person has into his or her values, beliefs, strengths and weaknesses. Inherent in the application of the principle of integrity is the principle of honesty and truth-telling (Thiroux, 1980; Seedhouse, 1988).

The practical face of integrity in action in the nurse who is undertaking research is in the guidelines outlined below.

In the practice of integrity, nurse researchers must:

- be aware of their own level of knowledge and skill, compared to the knowledge and skill required to undertake the research;
- refrain from carrying out research if the nature of that research is beyond the limits of their own abilities.

Both of these guidelines are a direct reflection of the UKCC *Code of Professional Conduct* (1992), which states that in exercising professional accountability, the nurse must:

> acknowledge any limitations in . . . knowledge and competence and decline any duties or responsibilities unless able to perform them in a safe and skilled manner.

This does not preclude nurses who are new to research

ing such research. Instead, integrity is about being the need for seeking and using supervision from an experienced researcher. This is not only an issue of integrity, but also one of responsibility to one's subjects, which will be discussed later in this chapter.

Knowing one's research limitations and seeking guidance and supervision from an experienced researcher is also a mechanism by which professional standards and credibility are maintained (RCN, 1993).

Researchers must also:

- be aware of their own subjectivity and any biases that could influence their research.

Bias is defined by Macleod-Clark and Hockey (1989) as:

distortion of the findings resulting from an undesirable influence.

In terms of integrity, researcher bias is the undesirable influence that can occur when the researcher's subjectivity influences the way she or he perceives, records and interprets research data. In terms of practising integrity as a researcher, the nurse needs to recognise potential prejudices and bias, and build ways of minimising bias into the research.

Furthermore, the nurse needs to:

- make available the results of research, including details of methodology, research tools and positive and negative data, as well as identifying the limitations of the research and the extent to which findings can be generalised.

Here, integrity is honesty and truth-telling made manifest. It is also part of exercising professional accountability as a researcher.

In making public all aspects of the research method and results, the nurse researcher also needs to:

- acknowledge when the work of others has been used, including gaining permission for the use of other people's research tools and adhering to copyright regulations.

Within this guideline for good research practice there is an overlap between behaving legally (e.g. adhering to copyright law) and behaving with integrity (the practice being ethical and demonstrating integrity).

Plagiarism is defined (Concise Oxford Dictionary, 1976) as:

taking and using another person's thoughts as one's own.

Avoiding plagiarism is a demonstration of professional integrity on the part of the researcher.

A final issue of integrity for nurses who undertake research is about seeking ethical approval. Nurse researchers should:

- present a formal written research proposal to an appropriate ethics committee, identifying any ethical implications of the research and seeking ethical approval.

This often presents problems to nurses who are undertaking research. The Royal College of Physicians (1990a) have published guidelines on the practice of ethics committees in medical research involving human subjects. It is common practice for these guidelines to be used by hospital ethics committees when scrutinising research proposals from doctors (and others) wishing to undertake clinical trials. It is also an expectation by the Royal College of Physicians (1990b) for all doctors undertaking clinical trials to seek ethical approval from a hospital or university ethics committee.

What is not common practice is for nurses to gain ethical approval from hospital ethics committees prior to undertaking their nursing research. There are several suggested reasons for this:

- A lack of knowledge and understanding on the part of nurse researchers as to the nature and importance of ethical scrutiny of a research proposal.
- A lack of appropriate criteria on the part of ethics committees to scrutinise nursing research proposals.

    Clinical trials by doctors (and others) have agreed criteria or frameworks against which a judgement can be made about the ethical issues within that proposal. These criteria are based on a 'risk-benefit' analysis (Castles, 1987; Royal College of Physicians, 1990b). Risk-benefit analysis is the operationalisation of two of the ethical principles underpinning medical ethics: beneficence and non-maleficence. In a clinical blind or double-blind trial, using experimental methodologies, risk-benefit analysis is indeed appropriate and is philosophically in tune with the principles underpinning medical ethics.

    However, nursing ethics, as argued throughout this chapter, needs to rely on other principles, and, therefore, criteria or frameworks appropriate to ethical principles in nursing ethics need to be created. In addition to this, the majority of nursing research studies do not use experimental methodologies, so appropriate methods for undertaking ethical scrutiny of qualitative and action research methodologies need to be sought.

- A lack of recognition on the part of many hospital ethics committees of the need for nursing research to come under their scrutiny.

This may be due partly to non-recognition of qualitative or action research methodology and partly to the medical and masculine dominance of many ethics committees and the historical undervaluing of nursing as a scientific, research–based, intellectual discipline.

Responsibility of nurse researchers to their subjects

Several key areas of ethical concern arise when examining the responsibility that researchers have to their subjects. Yet, in a wider sense, a discussion about the nurse researcher's responsibility to her or his subjects is also an extension of the principle of integrity.

Integrity with regard to the subjects within a nursing research study begins with an examination of the need for carrying out the study. The RCN (1993) states quite simply that prior to undertaking research, the nurse must be sure that the knowledge being sought is not already available. This is reinforced by the British Paediatric Association (1991), which states that research on children should not be carried out if the knowledge can be gained through comparable research on adults.

This statement can raise questions about what is the difference — in ethical terms — between research on children and research on adults. Is it that it is easier to ensure informed consent from adults? Is it because children have more rights than adults? Or is it because ethical behaviour is perhaps different towards adults than towards children? Do nurse researchers have different responsibilities with regard to children than to adults? What about research on other vulnerable groups, such as the elderly mentally ill or people with learning difficulties? Does responsibility — as a component of the ethical principle of integrity or conscience — mean different things to different groups of subjects?

The overriding notion of responsibility with regard to all research subjects is embodied in the following guidelines for good research practice:

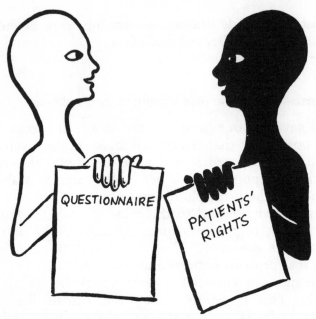

- Protect the research subject from any physical, emotional, mental, social or spiritual harm.
- If any harm, or possible harm, is anticipated, subjects should be warned of this in order to decide whether or not they wish to participate in the research.

As described previously, medical research that employs experimental design is scrutinised using a risk-benefit analysis. For nursing research, particularly research using qualitative, non-experimental approaches, such an analysis is impossible to undertake and yields little useful information upon which to make an ethical judgement of the research. Roach (1987) might instead ask, 'Does the research promote and demonstrate caring?' Johnstone (1989) might ask, 'Does the research recognise that patients (as people) have intrinsic moral worth? Am I respecting my subjects as autonomous choosers? Am I behaving as a researcher in such a way as to facilitate and support their choice?'

The responsibility of the nurse researcher to her or his subjects (whether the subjects are patients, clients, colleagues or others) can also be examined in terms of the principle of fidelity. Fidelity has been defined as trust or, put another way, faithfulness or loyalty. In practising fidelity to research subjects, the nurse researcher recognises that the relationship between researcher and subjects is based on the subjects' belief that the researcher will safeguard their interests. In practical terms, the nurse researcher demonstrates this through the following practices:

- Giving full and honest information to all research subjects about the nature of the research and its purpose, why they have been selected for inclusion in the study and how this selection was made, what they need to do or what will be done to them in the course of being a subject, and that ethical approval has been given.

  All this information should be given, both verbally and in writing, in terms and language that the subjects can understand.
- Giving subjects (especially patients or clients) verbal and written assurances that they can refuse to participate and can withdraw from being a subject at any time and that refusal or withdrawal will not jeopardise the care they receive.
- Giving assurances that all health and other related information obtained during the research is confidential, and gaining permission from subjects to use such information.
- Seeking consent by proxy from an appropriate advocate or significant other in the case of subjects unable to give consent (e.g. unconscious or mentally impaired clients, or children under school age) (BPA, 1991; RCN, 1993).

It may be of value to examine at this time the nature of the actual or potential role conflict between the nurse as a care-giver and the nurse as researcher. The nurse who is undertaking research also holds knowledge, skill and expertise in care-giving and may, in the course of undertaking research, feel that it is in the patient's interests (e.g. to uphold the patient's safety) to move into the care-giver role. It may be worth exploring in advance some key principles of this role duality, for example:

- what the differences are between the two roles and when role conflict might potentially arise;
- how any foreseeable role conflict might be resolved.

Relationships with sponsors, employers and colleagues

Much of the literature related to ethics and nursing research focuses primarily on nurses' responsibility to their subjects (Scott, 1982; Castles, 1987). However, the RCN (1993) recognises that nurse researchers also have ethical responsibilities to those who sponsor their research, those who employ them and colleagues.

Sponsors and employers

Although the ethical principle of integrity has been discussed earlier, the notion of responsibility to those who sponsor, commission or employ a nurse to undertake research is also concerned with the integrity of the researcher (see chapter 3). It is only the application of the principle of integrity that takes on different dimensions when the relationship between the researcher and sponsor or employer is under discussion. Just as nurses are required by the UKCC (1992) to acknowledge any limitation in competence and to decline any duties that they cannot perform safely and competently, so, too, the nurse researcher must do the same in a research context, for example because of being unable to undertake competently the research owing to insufficient time, money, people or equipment. Integrity on the part of the researcher is also related to clarifying to sponsors and/or employers that it is not possible to guarantee solutions to nursing problems, yet at the same time, to make clear in the research proposal what problems the research is attempting to find solutions for.

Researchers must also be clear about the conditions under which any grant or research funding is being given and what constraints, if any, are conditions of the award or grant being given. This is the practical side of honesty and entering into a fiduciary (trusting) relationship with sponsors and/or employers.

An extension of the discussion of role conflict in the previous section is about clarifying with employers when the nurse is in a care-giving role (and, therefore, has service responsibilities) and when she or he is in the research role. The nurse who is exclusively in a research role needs, as part of a relationship of trust, to clarify that she or he has no service-giving responsibility unless a subject requires protection or assistance from danger or harm. Scott (1982) highlights the ethical role of those who sponsor research and cites the sponsors' role in ensuring patient safety, ethical approval and provision of adequate resources.

Colleagues

In a research context, the colleagues of a nurse researcher include nurses, students and other health care professionals, including doctors. The principle of respecting persons equally (Seedhouse, 1988) and the principle of individual freedom (Thiroux, 1980) have very practical importance to the nurse researchers. Just as consent from patients is an ethical requirement of researchers, so consent from colleagues to participate in a nurse researcher's project must also be sought, although not necessarily in a formal, written way as from the research subjects. Researchers must be sensitive to the potential for exploitation inherent in unequal relationships. Informed consent from subjects ensures that the researcher does not coerce the subject into participation in the research. However, students and less senior nursing colleagues are also vulnerable to pressure from researchers to act as data collectors or to participate in some way in the research. This notion will also be revisited later in the chapter.

Historically, many nurses have perceived that, for any nursing research to be undertaken, permission must first be granted by the patient's consultant or general practitioner. It is now widely accepted that although some research may require some prior permission, much nursing research falls completely within the discipline of nursing and no such permission is required.

Autonomy implies that people should be free to choose and be entitled to act on their preferences, provided their decisions and actions do not stand to *violate or impinge on* the *moral* interests of others (Johnstone, 1989). Thus, a nurse undertaking research may choose, out of professional courtesy, to ensure that the consultant or general practitoner is aware that one of his or her patients is participating in a nursing research study. However, if the doctor's *moral* interests are not being infringed, the nurse researcher can act autonomously in the research study.

Nurses in Positions of Authority in Research Settings

Five particular ethical principles can be applied to nurses who are in positions of authority where research is being carried out. These are:

- justice or fairness;
- individual freedom;
- honesty or truth-telling;
- trust;
- confidentiality.

Justice or fairness

This principle, described by Thiroux (1980) and Rawls (1973), is related to equal distribution. Thiroux speaks of equal distribution in terms of distribution of good and bad, while Rawls described equal distribution in terms of distribution of resources.

The nurse in a position of authority where research is to be carried out must be satisfied that the research is 'worthwhile', 'good' or being done for 'good' and that it is achievable. Her or his responsibility also extends to making decisions as to the extent to which the research project is feasible in terms of service demands and available resources.

Individual freedom

Any nurse who is in a position to commission research or employ a nurse researcher must also respect the researcher's right to refuse to undertake the commission if, in the researcher's view, the research is outside her or his competence or is not feasible due to resource constraints. Respecting individuals' freedom is also about avoiding coercion or pressure within the hierarchical relationship on a nurse researcher to carry out such research if she or he feels unable to do so.

Honesty or truth-telling, trust and confidentiality

A nurse who commissions a research study must respect all promises of confidentiality given to subjects by the researcher. The nurse in a position of authority, as part of the trust which she or he is ascribed by others, needs to avoid probing data or research results in order to try to identify the individual subjects who supplied the data.

This is perhaps most applicable in research projects in which other nurses are the subjects and data is being collected from nurses themselves. The confidentiality assured by the researcher must be respected by the nurse in a position of authority, and in no way should any attempt be made to identify the source of the data or to use it for punitive or disciplinary actions.

There is an ethical tension between the professional obligation on the part of a nurse manager to facilitate research wherever possible, both to advance the profession and to ensure quality care delivery, and the obligation to ensure that the interests of patients, staff and the service are not compromised by the demands of research being undertaken.

Involvement of Nurses in Other People's Research

It is in this sphere that nurses can experience conflict between their role as nurse practitioners and their role as participants or helpers in research being undertaken by other nurses or health care professionals.

As practitioners, there are two main areas of ethical responsibility. The first of these is related to the role of ensuring that free and informed consent has been obtained from patients or clients prior to their involvement as subjects within a research project. Practising nurses, therefore, have a responsibility to understand what informed consent means and to be conversant with the principles and procedures for obtaining informed consent, and they should satisfy themselves that prior to consenting to be a subject within a research study, the client or patient understands what it will mean to be a subject, what it will entail and any possible adverse effects of participating. This responsibility is part of a nurse's role as patient advocate, an ethical concept described by Gadow (1983), Curtin (1986) and Marks-Maran (1993a).

The second area of ethical responsibility is about whistleblowing, applied to misuse of the research process. Each nurse has a responsibility to ensure that research is conducted ethically (RCN, 1993). Whistleblowing as an ethical response to errors, negligence or mistreatment of clients can be traced back to 1910 when the American Journal of Nursing published an editorial on the subject (*American Journal of Nursing*, 1910).

Bok (1986) wrote that:

> the alarm of the whistleblower is meant to disrupt the status quo: to pierce the background noise, perhaps the false harmony, or the imposed silence of 'business as usual'.

Whistleblowing in health care has come to be associated with reporting poor standards of practice or adequate resources not being made available for the minimal level of acceptable care.

In a research context, nurses may find themselves working in clinical areas in which other people are carrying out research and where they perhaps observe unethical practice related to that research. This might be absence of consent being sought for subjects' participation, patients being left untreated, or the service to patients or clients being adversely affected by the amount of time and resources being put into the research, to the detriment of overall patient care. In such cases, nurses have a reponsibility to ensure that all research is carried out in an ethical way (RCN, 1993) and should (UKCC, 1992):

> report to an appropriate person or authority any circumstances in which safe and appropriate care for patients and clients cannot be provided.

As data collectors for other people's research, nurses also have ethical responsibilities and potential dilemmas. Within the ethical principle of justice or fairness (Rawls, 1973; Thiroux, 1980), there is an ethical issue surrounding the amount of time and effort expected of a nurse as a data collector for someone else's research versus the time required to provide care to patients. The RCN (1993) states that nurses have an obligation to make it known to appropriate people if the extra responsibility as a data collector might, or has, become detrimental to their normal work.

The principle of integrity, with regard to honesty and accuracy in the way in which data are collected and recorded, also applies to nurses who are acting as data collectors.

The issue of confidentiality is also one requiring discussion within the dual role of the nurse as researcher and the nurse as practitioner. There will be occasions when the nurse obtains information from the patient as part of her or his role as care-giver. This information is confidential to the care-giving team and, unless agreed by the patient (subject) beforehand, cannot be made available to the research team. Conversely, information collected as part of the data collection role is confidential to the research team. As such, the nurse is unable within the ethics of confidentiality to use this information in the course of her or his role as practitioner without first gaining permission from the leader of the research, who in turn must gain this permission from the research subjects (RCN, 1993).

One final area of potential ethical conflict can occur when nurses are involved as data collectors in commercially sponsored research. As with all other research, nurses must satisfy themselves that the research is ethically sound but, in line with the UKCC *Code of Professional Conduct* (1992), should:

> ensure that [their] registration status is not used in the promotion of commercial products or services, declare any financial or other interests in relevant organisations providing such goods or services and ensure that [their] professional judgement is not influenced by commercial considerations.

Using (or not Using) Research Findings in Nursing Practice

One purpose of undertaking research is to advance nursing knowledge to improve patient care. Brykczyńska (1989) makes the point that 'nursing research activity . . . must have an ethical value'. She cites badly designed research, incorrectly conducted research or research that violates the principles of beneficence as examples of breaking the 'covenant' between researcher and patient. The covenant here is the advocacy — or trust — relationship between nurse (researcher) and patient. Therefore, a requirement of undertaking research is to uphold the principle of good or right (Thiroux, 1980) in terms of patients.

A second purpose of undertaking research is to benefit the nursing profession (Brykczyńska, 1989). Macleod-Clark and Hockey (1979) wrote:

> In some ways it is often the simplest procedures that are most in need of scrutiny, for these are the aspects of nursing practice which are taken for granted and have become firmly incorporated into the routinised fabric of nursing.

Walsh and Ford (1989) reiterated this by demonstrating

that nursing care is failing the patient because it is insti-tution-driven rather than patient-driven, and suggest that the cause of this failure is rooted in traditional rituals and myths. They define ritual as undertaking a task without thinking it through in a problem-solving, logical way, and demonstrate that much of nursing care today is ritualised and inappropriate care, despite the presence of a wide range of research studies offering ways of carrying out care that have been demonstrated to be more therapeutic and beneficial to patients. Walsh and Ford ask the question 'Why should a profession behave so unprofessionally?'. However, the question perhaps ought to be 'Why should a profession behave so unethically?'

Roach (1987) might suggest that the ethical 'rightness' of a nursing action is that it is the most caring action. Her five C's (above) attempted to define what is meant by caring. One of these — competence — is particularly relevant when examining the implications of not using research findings in practice. Competence has earlier been defined as the state of having the experience, skill, judge-ment and wisdom to respond appropriately. Judgement and wisdom in nursing are about making choices that are in the interests of patient care, and, as such, choosing appropriate research-based actions is inherent in judge-ment and wisdom. One can only conclude that to make choices for nursing practice that do not reflect research findings demonstrates poor judgement and lack of wisdom and, therefore, lack of competence. If there is no com-petence, there is inappropriate, or inadequate, caring.

The UKCC (1992) states that in the exercise of pro-fessional accountability the nurse shall:

> Maintain and improve . . . professional knowledge and competence.

The UKCC offers standards of professional practice in the form of the statements within the *Code of Professional Conduct*.

They are within the scope of accountability in that any nurse may, at any time, be called upon to justify her or his nursing actions (and therefore her or his nursing judgement).

Accountability (Burnard and Chapman, 1988; Marks-Maran, 1993b) is defined as being answerable for or having to justify one's actions. Professional practice demands that in justifying or answering for nursing judgements and nursing actions, nurses are expected to demonstrate that they keep up to date with nursing knowledge and nursing research to guide those judgements and actions. But accountability is not just a professional issue. There is also, as described earlier, legal accountability (being answerable to the law), managerial accountability (being answerable to management) and moral accountability (being answerable to one's conscience or a defined or articulated set of ethical principles). It is possible for a person to experience conflict between all of these, and what one truly believes to be good or right (moral accountability) can be in conflict with what is deemed to be either professionally, managerially or legally right (Marks–Maran 1993b).

Use of research to base nursing judgements and actions on is a professional expectation, but it may not be a managerial or legal expectation. The question for each nurse must be 'Is it a moral expectation?'. If using research findings and engaging in research-based practice is seen as a moral expectation — based on the ethical principles of good or right (Thiroux, 1980) or beneficence (Beauchamp and Childress, 1983) — *not* to use research in practice can only be seen as acting immorally.

Conclusions

Ethical issues, questions and dilemmas arise in all spheres of nursing practice; it would be short-sighted to assume that nursing research is exempt from this.

This chapter has attempted to take the reader through a process of examining ethical issues in nursing research, starting with an exploration of the relationship between ethical principles and nursing research and then critically applying these ethical principles to four particular areas of nursing research activity: nurses who carry out research, nurses in positions of authority where research is being carried out, nurses who work in areas where other professionals are carrying out research, and the ethical implications of using (or not using) research in nursing practice.

Two themes have influenced the writing of this chapter, firstly, that nursing ethics is distinct and separate from medical ethics and may be underpinned by different ethical principles from those underpinning medical ethics, and secondly, that ethical deliberation is a personal moral journey as well as a professional one.

Brykczyńska (1989) wrote:

> Nurses must reach the stage at which nursing research is an inseparable component of the practice process. . . .

Perhaps the real message of this chapter is that nurses must reach the stage at which practising *ethically* is inseparable from undertaking research and engaging in nursing care.

References

American Journal of Nursing (1910) Where does loyalty end?. *American Journal of Nursing*, 10: pp. 230–1.

Beauchamp T and Childress J (1983) *Principles of Biomedical Ethics* (2nd edn.). Oxford: Oxford University Press.

Benjamin M and Curtis J (1986) *Ethics in Nursing* (2nd edn.). New York: Oxford University Press.

Bok S (1978) *Lying: Moral Choice in Public and Private Life.* New York: Random House.

Bok S (1986) *Secrets: Concealment and Revelation.* New York: Oxford University Press.

British Paediatric Association (1991) *Guidelines for the Ethical Conduct of Research Involving Children.* Unpublished document.

Brykczyńska G (1989) Ethics of nursing research: ethical implications of not undertaking research and for ignoring results of research. *International Journal of Medicine & Law,* 8 (2): pp. 199–204.

Burnard P and Chapman C (1988) *Professional and Ethical Issues in Nursing.* Chichester: John Wiley and Sons.

Castles M R (1987) *A Primer of Nursing Research.* Philadelphia: W B Saunders.

Concise Oxford Dictionary (1976) J B Sykes (ed.). *Dictionary of Current English.* Oxford: Oxford University Press.

Curtin L (1986) The nurse as an advocate: a philosophical foundation for nursing. In P L Chinn (ed.) *Ethical Issues in Nursing.* Germantown, Maryland: Aspen Publications.

Davis A and Aroskar M (1983) *Ethical Dilemmas and Nursing Practice* (2nd edn.). Norwalk, Connecticut: Appleton Century Crofts.

Flaherty M J (1982) Nursing's contract with society. In L Curtin and M J Flaherty (eds) *Nursing Ethics: Theories and Pragmatics.* Bowie, Maryland: Robert J Brady.

Gadow S (1983) Existential advocacy: philosophical foundations of nursing. In C D Murphy and H Hunter (eds) *Ethical Problems in the Nurse–Patient Relationship.* Boston, Massachusetts: Allyn and Bacon.

Gilligan C (1987) Moral orientation and moral development. In E Kittay and D Meyers (eds) *Women and Moral Theory.* Totowa, New Jersey: Rowman and Littlefield.

Gillon R (1986) *Philosophical Medical Ethics.* Chichester: John Wiley and Sons.

Johnstone M J (1987) Ethics in focus. *The Australian Nurses Journal,* 17 (3): pp. 41–2.

Johnstone M J (1989) *Bioethics: A Nursing Perspective.* Marrickville, NSW: W B Saunders.

Kant I (1972) *The Moral Law* (translated by H J Paton). London: Hutchinson University Library.

Kohlberg L (1981) *The Philosophy of Moral Development: Moral Stages and the Idea of Justice.* San Francisco: Harper and Row.

Macleod–Clark J and Hockey L (1979) *Research For Nursing: a Guide for the Enquiring Nurse*. Aylesbury: HM & M.

Macleod–Clark J and Hockey L (1989) *Further Research for Nursing*. London: Scutari Press.

Marks–Maran D (1993a) Advocacy. In V Tschudin (ed.) *Ethics: Nurses and Patients*. London: Scutari Press.

Marks–Maran D (1993b) Accountability. In V Tschudin (ed.) *Ethics: Nurses and Patients*. London: Scutari Press.

Mayeroff M (1971) *On Caring*. New York: Harper and Row.

Melia K M (1989) *Everyday Nursing Ethics*. Basingstoke: Macmillan.

Niebuhr H R (1963) *The Responsible Self*. San Francisco: Harper and Row.

Nouwen H J M (1982) *Compassion*. London: Darton, Longman and Todd.

Rawls J (1973) *A Theory of Justice*. Oxford: Oxford University Press.

Roach M S (1987) *The Human Act of Caring*. Ottawa: Canadian Hospitals Association.

Royal College of Nursing (1993) *Ethics Related to Research* (2nd edn.). London: RCN.

Royal College of Physicians (1990a) *Guidelines on the Practice of Ethics Committees in Medical Research Involving Human Subjects*. London: Royal College of Physicians.

Royal College of Physicians (1990b) *Research Involving Patients*. London: Royal College of Physicians.

Rumbold G (1986) *Ethics in Nursing Practice*. London: Baillière Tindall.

Scott D (1982) Ethical issues in nursing research: access to human subjects. *Topics in Clinical Nursing*, April, pp. 78–83.

Seedhouse D (1988) *Ethics: The Heart of Health Care*. Chichester: John Wiley and Sons.

Thiroux J P (1980) *Ethics: Theory and Practice* (2nd edn.). Encino, California: Glencoe Publishing.

Thompson I E, Melia K and Boyd K (1983) *Nursing Ethics*. Edinburgh: Churchill Livingstone.

Tschudin V (1992) *Ethics in Nursing: The Caring Relationship* (2nd edn.) Oxford: Butterworth-Heinemann.

Tschudin V and Marks–Maran D (1993) *Ethics: A primer for*

nurses. Workbook and workshop guide. London: Baillière Tindall.

UKCC (1992) *Code of Professional Conduct* (3rd edn.). London: UKCC.

Veatch R M (1985) Nursing ethics, physician ethics and medical ethics. *Bioethics Reporter*, 6/7: pp. 381–3.

Walsh M and Ford P (1989) *Nursing Rituals: Research and Rational Action*. Oxford: Butterworth-Heinemann.

CHAPTER 3

Research Ethics Committees

Barbara Parker

Nursing is said to have 'come of age' when it started its own research. To advance nursing as a profession, and to advance in their careers, nurses have to be research-oriented. This means contact with research ethics committees (RECs).

In this chapter the author, the secretary of a research ethics committee, outlines with great clarity how RECs work and what they require. This chapter will be most helpful not only to anyone considering research, but also to readers concerned with the development of ethics and research and those who are asked to participate in research, either as subjects or colleagues. The detailed information given will help nurses at all levels, not least in the development of their advocacy role.

Research Ethics Committees (RECs) exist because of a need to ensure that research involving human subjects is not only conducted ethically, but also seen to be ethical. Researchers have a moral obligation to conduct ethical research, but it is generally considered that they should not be the sole judge of this and that proposed research projects should be subject to independent ethical review.

Nurses, Nursing Research and RECs

In the course of their work, nurses are likely to come into contact with the work of RECs on three levels:

- as nurses who are required to assist in the implemen-

tation of research protocols during the course of performing their everyday duties;
- as researchers seeking ethical approval of a research project;
- as nurse members of an REC.

The participation of nurses in implementing research initiated by others is vital: without them, the vast majority of studies, many of which are extremely nursing-intensive, would not take place.

The UKCC's *Code of Professional Conduct* (1992) states that:

> As a registered nurse, midwife or health visitor, you are personally accountable for your practice.

It goes on to say that, in exercising such accountability, it is necessary to:

> maintain and improve your professional knowledge and competence.

Hence, nurses are increasingly initiating and carrying out their own research. For these reasons, nurses must be aware of the ethical issues relating to research involving human beings and of the work of RECs in maintaining ethical standards.

Much nursing research is qualitative in nature, and there have been criticisms that such work is not well understood by RECs. It has been suggested that there is a need to consider whether or not nursing research should be 'reviewed by a separately constituted nursing review committee, as in parts of North America' (Hunt, 1992). Such a move could have the effect of 'side-lining' the valuable research undertaken by nurses, and, in order for nursing research to achieve appropriate status, it is important that it should continue to be considered alongside medical research proposals. What is needed is more care in the selection and appointment of REC members generally,

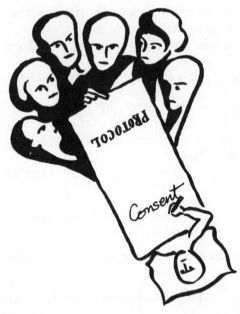

including the appointment of more nurses of an appropriate calibre and experience, and adequate training for all members of RECs to enable them better to understand and value nursing research.

As members of RECs, nurses have much to offer, and the importance of the potential contribution that they can make should not be underestimated. Nurses are uniquely placed not only to have a full understanding of the purpose and nature of the research proposed, but also to have a special insight into the day-to-day implications that participating in a clinical research project can have for the research subject.

History and Development of RECs

Public interest and concern about the ethics of research involving human subjects came to the fore following revelations about the experimentation conducted under Nazi rule, but it was not until 1964 that the World Medical Association, at its 18th World Medical Assembly in Helsinki, adopted *Recommendations Guiding Physicians in Biomedical Research Involving Human Subjects*, known as the Declaration of Helsinki. These recommendations were subsequently amended in 1975, 1983 and, most recently, 1989 by the 41st World Medical Assembly in Hong Kong and remain the most authoritative guide for researchers and those participating in ethical review. The second 'basic principle' of these recommendations states that protocols should be formulated for experimental procedures involving human subjects and that these should be submitted:

> to a specially appointed committee independent of the investigator and the sponsor provided that this independent committee is in conformity with the laws and regulations of the country in which the research experiment is performed.

In 1967, not long after the Surgeon-General of the USA ruled that institutions accepting federal funds should establish independent ethical review of research proposals, the Royal College of Physicians of London recommended that clinical research proposals should be subject to ethical review. Following this, the Ministry of Health issued a memorandum indicating that health authorities should organise ethical review on an informal and advisory basis.

RECs are now to be found in most health districts and trusts, although, in view of a lack of authoritative guidance over a long period, there has been great disparity in their structure and conduct and confusion as to their role and the scope of their responsibilities and powers.

RECs and the Law

It is interesting to note that, in England, there has never been a statute specifically regulating the conduct of research on human subjects, although there is one for animals. In law, there is no obligation placed upon an institution to establish an REC, nor is there a formal legal requirement for researchers to submit their proposed research project for ethical review.

However, in its Executive Summary, the Department of Health's (DoH) health service guidelines *Local Research Ethics Committees* (1991) state that:

> Every health district should have a local research ethics committee (LREC) to advise NHS bodies on the ethical acceptability of research proposals involving human subjects.

It goes on to direct that:

> Any NHS body asked to agree a research proposal falling within its sphere of responsibility should ensure that it has been submitted to the appropriate LREC for research ethics approval

but makes it clear that:

> Responsibility for deciding whether a research proposal should proceed, within the NHS, lies with the NHS body under whose auspices the research would take place

and that the RECs, should not be regarded as a 'management arm' of the constituting authority.

Although there is no legal requirement to implement these guidelines, the remit of which is limited to the NHS in England, the authority wielded by RECs is considerable, and researchers working within the NHS will not have access to its patients without ethical approval of the proposed research. Additionally, those bodies which fund research usually require the proposal to have been approved by an REC and, increasingly, without such approval, the results of the research may not be published.

Objectives of RECs

The objectives of RECs have been defined by the Royal College of Physicians (RCP) in its *Guidelines on the Practice of Ethics Committees in Medical Research Involving Human Subjects* (1990a) as being:

> to maintain ethical standards of practice in research, to protect subjects of research from harm, to preserve the subjects' rights and to provide reassurance to the public that this is being done.

In meeting these objectives, RECs should seek to facilitate and promote good ethical research and not to stand in the way of research work that will be of benefit to society. As a by-product of meeting such objectives, RECs should also be available to offer sound research ethics advice to those seeking to undertake research involving human subjects and will protect researchers from any unjustified allegations of unethical practice.

RECs have no remit to consider ethical issues relating to clinical practice generally. Indeed, the RCP guidelines state that:

> Research Ethics Committees are not currently constituted for this purpose and it is unwise of a Committee to respond formally to requests that are outside its terms of reference.

This would appear to be reinforced by the DoH (1991), which has included the word 'research' in the title of its health service guidelines *Local Research Ethics Committees*.

There has been much discussion about the need for a national ethics committee and the role such a body might play. It has been variously suggested that it should be responsible for overseeing the work of local RECs, setting standards, initiating training for REC members and having an involvement in the ethical review of multicentre research. Perhaps the consideration of ethical issues relating to general clinical practice should more appropriately be undertaken by such a body.

Membership of RECs

The calibre of an REC and the quality of the research ethics advice that it offers the researcher will depend, to a very great extent, on the selection of members with the appropriate knowledge, background and personal qualities. The RCP, in its guidelines (1990a), considers that members of RECs:

> need to be people of goodwill, with a high regard for the human personality, for truthfulness and for the continued advance of science in the interest of society

and goes on to say that:

> individuals who are acquiescent and may be thought likely to give automatic approval are also not suitable members.

There is no set formula for the composition of RECs, and the size of a committee and the backgrounds of individual members may depend, to some extent, on the nature of the research that the REC is required to review and the working practices and procedures it has adopted. Lay members, nurses and general practitioner members of RECs have a particular responsibility to look at a research project from the point of view of the research subject. Nurse members of RECs will be concerned to ensure that any proposed research will not have a detrimental effect on the care a patient receives.

The DoH health service guidelines (1991) lay down a number of requirements for membership of RECs: RECs must have from eight to 12 members, of both sexes, who are drawn from a wide range of age groups; they should include hospital medical and nursing staff, general practitioners and two or more lay people, and either the chair or the vice-chair of the REC must be a lay person.

Members should be people of good judgement and appropriate background and experience, and it is important to be aware that, although they may be drawn from groups having specific interests or responsibilities in connection with health care, REC members serve not as representatives of those groups, but as people in their own right.

In *Ethics and Health Care, The Role of Research Ethics Committees in the United Kingdom* (1992), Neuberger examined the work of RECs in the UK. She found that while the majority of RECs surveyed conformed to guidelines, the membership of a 'substantial minority' differed in at least one or more respects. For example, while most of the committees surveyed had at least one nurse member, some 12 per cent had none and only 7 per cent had two or more. Women and ethnic minorities were poorly represented.

Of particular concern is that one third of the committees surveyed had fewer than the minimum number of lay members recommended by the DoH. One difficulty is that there is no clear definition of exactly what constitutes a 'lay' member. For example, some would consider a member of the clergy or even a nurse to be a lay member. Can an officer of the health authority or trust which has constituted an REC and who serves as a member of the committee truly be considered a lay member? Conversely, is the well-intentioned person in the street, who may have no previous knowledge of or training in medical or ethical matters, able to make an appropriate contribution to the work of an REC?

Whatever the 'skill-mix' of an REC, it is clearly important that individual members should not feel outnumbered or overawed by their fellow members and should not be constrained from expressing their opinions and concerns.

Working Practices and Procedures of RECs

As with the membership of RECs, the working practices and procedures of individual committees may vary considerably and may, to a certain extent, be dependent on the quantity and nature of the research proposals that have to be considered. The DoH (1991) guidelines require that standing orders setting out the frequency of meetings and the working methods of RECs be drawn up by the constituting body, and that situations in which the chair's action may be taken are clearly described. The RCP guidelines give more detailed guidance on the working practices and procedures of RECs. Both the DoH and the RCP guidelines strongly discourage the conduct of REC business by post or telephone, although some committees may still work in this way. Applicants should be aware that they may be required to attend an REC meeting to present their proposal in person and discuss it with the committee. This can be a positive and valuable learning experience both for the researcher and the REC.

Monitoring the Progress of Approved Projects and Enforcing REC Recommendations

The responsibility of an REC does not cease with the approval or non-approval of a project, and RECs should monitor the progress of the projects that they have approved in an attempt to ensure that their conduct remains ethical, particularly in the light of any proposed significant deviations from the originol protocol or of any unusual or unexpected results that may raise concerns about the continued safety of the research. Given that an REC's primary objective is to protect the research subject, it should also take steps to ensure that the rights of the research subject are being maintained, particularly with regard to recruitment, information and consent procedures. More generally, in seeking feedback with regard to the progress of approved projects, RECs may obtain valuable information that can be taken into account when considering future applications.

Neuberger (1992) considers that there is a growing awareness among REC members of the requirement for RECs to undertake a monitoring role, but in her study many chairpersons of RECs believed that this was beyond their resources, while others did not see it as an appropriate role for RECs. Even when a formal monitoring system has been introduced, it can be of only limited value unless the REC is able effectively to use the information that is generated and take appropriate action if there is concern that ethical standards are not, for whatever reason, being maintained. The RCP (1990a) suggests that:

> Where a Committee is dissatisfied with the conduct of an investigation it may withdraw approval already given.

RECs have no direct sanctions, but in its guidelines (1991), the DoH says that if it comes to the attention of an REC that research that has not been submitted for ethical approval is being undertaken, or that its recommendations are not being adhered to, the REC is required to report the matter to its appointing authority and any appropriate professional body. Researchers should be aware that they could be subject to professional disciplinary or legal proceedings if they fail to seek or ignore the advice of an REC.

At a time of increasing public awareness of the rights of the individual, it is inevitable that interest in and awareness of the role and functions of RECs will intensify, and there is, more than ever, a need for research involving human subjects to be seen to be conducted ethically. It is, therefore, important that there should be clarification of the role of RECs in monitoring the research to which they have given ethical approval, and consistency in the application of sanctions against those who do not conform to the RECs' recommendations. The question of whether or not RECs should be given more authority in this respect remains to be addressed. It could be argued that if RECs were given more 'teeth', they would ensure that they were not bypassed or ignored by researchers.

Confidentiality of REC Proceedings and Accessibility of RECs

Both the DoH (1991) and the RCP (1990a) guidelines consider that the proceedings of REC meetings should remain confidential. The reasons given are that the issues considered may be complicated and delicate and that uninformed or unbalanced publicity may be damaging, especially to research subjects, that REC members do not serve as representatives of specific groups and need to be able to discuss the applications that come before them freely, and that, in the case of some applications, there will be a need to preserve commercial confidentiality.

However, both sets of guidelines recommend that an REC should submit an annual report to the authority or authorities that it advises and that this report should be made available for public inspection. Such a report should include names of committee members, details of the number of meetings held and the titles of the proposals considered, including whether or not they were approved and whether they were approved after amendment.

In practice, the attitude of RECs to publicity differs widely and is probably dictated, to a considerable extent, by the stance adopted by the authority or trust that the individual REC was constituted to advise. Neuberger's (1992) research indicated that few RECs issued a report that was in the public domain, although most produced reports for the health authorities that set them up. If RECs are to be seen to be effective in protecting the rights of the research subject, they and the authorities or trusts that constitute them may have to adopt a more open approach to publicity about their work. Should, for example, REC meetings be open to the public? This would assist RECs in fulfilling their objective of providing reassurance to the public that ethical standards of practice were being maintained, but could it also serve to raise undue anxiety in patients who may be invited to participate in the research under consideration?

In both its guidelines (1990a) and *Research Involving Patients* (1990b), the RCP makes it clear that research subjects who may be dissatisfied should be given access to the REC and that it is the responsibility of the investigator to make this known to research subjects. The question of how such access might be managed is not addressed, but it would be important to ensure that the grounds on which access to an REC was sought were appropriate and that in granting such access the patient–doctor–nurse relationship was not compromised.

Hospital staff, and nurses in particular, who may be required to participate in the implementation of research involving human subjects should also be able to feel free to raise any concerns that they may have about that research with the relevant REC; in fact, they have a duty to do so. The reality is that, in general, they do not, either because they are unaware that this is a possible course of action or because they are unwilling or feel unqualified to challenge the work of the researcher with whom they may have to maintain a good working relationship. Indeed, members of RECs themselves, including medical members, may feel constrained not to raise and pursue concerns about the work of their colleagues.

What Does or Does not Require Ethical Review?

According to the RCP (1990a) guidelines:

> All medical research involving human subjects should
> undergo ethical review before it commences, in
> accordance with the principle that investigators should not
> be the sole judge of whether their research raises significant
> ethical issues.

This includes both therapeutic and non-therapeutic research and work involving patients and healthy volunteers. The DoH (1991) advises that RECs must be consulted about all research projects involving NHS patients. This includes the use of fetal material and in vitro fertilisation, research on NHS premises involving the recently dead, access to the records of NHS patients and the use of or access to NHS facilities or premises.

It is left to the discretion of individual RECs to determine whether a project bearing minimal risk of distress or injury to the research subject might have less significant ethical implications and might, therefore, be considered less formally. There will be variation in practice from committee to committee.

The RCP (1990a) states that 'Ethical review is not required for studies that amount to quality control or medical audit'. This might include the collection or analysis of data in order to monitor the care provided to patients, but is subject to the proviso that the results of such work are not made available in a form that would compromise patient confidentiality.

There are difficulties about the definition of what constitutes medical research as distinct from medical practice. At what point does innovation become formal research? The RCP guidelines state that 'The distinction derives from the *intent*', in that in medical practice the sole intention is to obtain benefit to the individual patient while in medical research the main intention is to advance knowledge to the benefit of patients in general. The guidelines go on to say that when there is a significant departure from standard practice for the benefit of an individual patient with that patient's consent, this need not be regarded as research, but when this is extended into wider or more general use, it must be considered to be research.

One of the most common questions asked of an REC secretary is whether or not a piece of work requires ethical approval, and there is a need for more specific and detailed guidance on this. In the meantime, the golden rule must be — when in doubt, seek the advice of the REC.

Making an Application for Ethical Approval

Increasingly, nurses are undertaking research that will require the prior approval of an REC. The prospect of making an application for ethical approval, including, possibly, presenting the application in person to the committee, may appear daunting, particularly if it is for the first time. Nurses should remember, however, that the REC is there to assist them to undertake good ethical research by reviewing their proposal and offering sound research ethics advice.

Many RECs have now developed pro forma application documents, and the first step should be to contact the

secretary of the REC to which a submission will be made
in order to obtain a copy of the application form and to
find out as much as possible about the practices, procedures
and requirements of that committee, including the dates
of forthcoming meetings. This should be done as soon as
possible (even before the research protocol is written),
particularly if one is working to a tight schedule for the
completion of a project. A proforma application form may
be a useful guide to what information and documents the
REC will wish to have in order to consider an application.
Some RECs will also offer their own written guidelines
for the completion of the form. By making an early
approach to the REC in this way, it is possible to ensure
that all the necessary information has been assembled and
incorporated into the application and the research
protocol.

If applicants do not already know who the members of
the REC are, they should seek this information from the
secretary, since an awareness of the areas of expertise or
particular concerns of individual members of the committee may be helpful, in that it will be possible to ensure
that these topics are well covered in the application. The
secretary of the REC may also be able to advise on
whether individual members of the committee may be
approached for advice during the preparation of an application.

Before submitting an application, it will be necessary to
seek the written approval of the consultant (or general
practitioner in the case of non-hospital patients) who will
have overall responsibility for the research subjects whose
participation will be sought. The consultant should be
given the opportunity to scrutinise the research proposal,
including the application. Again, this will need to be dealt
with as early as possible, and RECs may wish to see formal
evidence that such approval has been given. Indeed, some
RECs may wish the consultant who will have overall

responsibility for the research subjects to bear ultimate responsibility for the research that is to be undertaken, and this will necessitate seeking his or her participation and cooperation in making the application. Applicants should also consult with colleagues and other groups who may be affected by the research they intend to carry out.

In preparing an application, it should be borne in mind that there is a need to ensure that an explanation of the project is given in lay terms, avoiding the use of medical jargon, which may not be readily understood by lay members of RECs.

Particular care should be taken in drawing up the proposed patient information sheet and consent form (see below), since these are considered to be of great importance by RECs and will, therefore, be subject to special scrutiny. Neuberger's (1992) research showed that, on average, some 35 per cent of information sheets are returned to the researcher to be rewritten and amendments are requested to a further 20 per cent.

Not only does the patient information sheet summarise the information that will be given to the potential research subject as part of the process of obtaining valid consent to participate in the research, but it also gives an indication to the REC of how well an applicant has thought through the implications and consequences of the study for the research subject. It is important to ensure that no information given in the patient information sheet conflicts with what is contained in either the application form or the protocol.

Some RECs will have a preferred consent form that applicants will be expected or advised to use. If this is not the case, applicants should draw up and submit for approval the form that they wish to use, taking care to see that the method by which they wish to obtain and record consent is appropriate to the nature of the research proposed.

Applicants should be aware that failure to fill in the application form correctly or completely, or to submit the necessary supporting documents, e.g. consent form, patient information sheet or letter to the general practitioner, could result in an application being rejected without consideration or the progress of an application being delayed.

Consideration of a Research Proposal by an REC

In order to consider whether or not a research proposal is acceptable on ethical grounds, and thereby fulfils its primary objective, the REC will wish to receive a considerable amount of information about the project, and this will be reflected in the application form. The information required may vary depending upon the nature of the project to be considered, but the following list is offered as a summary of the points upon which an REC will wish to satisfy itself.

- The researcher should be appropriately qualified and experienced to undertake the project. For example, it would clearly be wrong for a researcher to undertake a procedure on a patient for the purposes of research if she or he would not normally have been considered qualified to undertake that procedure as part of routine clinical management.
- The conditions under which the research is to be carried out must be suitable. For example, a patient being asked to respond to questions of an intimate nature would need to be assured of privacy. This would, of course, apply equally well in a situation where such questions were being asked for the purposes of routine clinical management.
- The project must be scientifically sound (in some

institutions it may be necessary for a project to be subjected to scientific review by a separate committee before it can be put forward for ethical consideration) and sufficient subjects need to be recruited to produce useful or valid results, although not more than are necessary to achieve this.

It would clearly be wrong to subject patients, even those with a life-threatening disease for whom no further active treatment was available, to a toxic drug with unpleasant side effects, unless there was a sound scientific basis for believing that the substance could be of benefit, nor would it be right to subject 50 patients to the drug when the inclusion of, say, 20 patients would be sufficient to determine whether or not it was of benefit.

- The proposed duration of the project should be compatible with the aims.
- Where appropriate (particularly in connection with studies involving healthy volunteers), the general practitioner responsible for a research subject should be contacted in connection with the patient's participation in the research, provided that the subject has consented to this. Should a research subject withhold such consent, he or she should be excluded from participation in the study.

The researcher has a responsibility to ensure that a potential research subject is fit to participate. For example, it is possible that a general practitioner may be aware of specific reasons why an individual patient might be particularly upset to receive a questionnaire that included questions about family or personal history of a hereditary disease. In certain circumstances, it might be important for a general practitioner to be aware of any study medication the participant is receiving in order to treat or prescribe for that patient appropriately if consulted on another or related matter.

- Patient confidentiality must be maintained. (Confidentiality will be discussed more fully later in this chapter.)
- The risks to the research subject must be justified, bearing in mind the aims of the project, both with regard to the care of the research subject and the advancement of knowledge generally. For example, in Auckland, New Zealand, women with carcinoma in situ of the cervix had (without their knowledge and, therefore, their consent) been included in a research project that had been formulated to demonstrate that their condition would not progress to a more invasive and more serious malignancy. As a consequence of their participation in this study, patients had been denied the treatment required to prevent the spread of their cancer (Campbell, 1989). In this case, whatever the aims of the project, they could not outweigh the risks to the individual.
- Any discomfort suffered by the subject as a consequence of the research should be no greater than necessary and commensurate with the intended benefit, and, in the case of non-therapeutic research, the risk to the research subject should be minimal. For example, it would not be appropriate to subject a healthy volunteer to radiation from repeated x-rays if the information required could be obtained from patients undergoing such investigations for the purposes of routine clinical management.
- Arrangements should be in place for compensating the research subject for any injury arising out of his or her participation in the research. In the case of research sponsored by private companies, the REC will need to satisfy itself that arrangements for compensation have adequate financial backing and that

the company accepts and will abide by the Association of the British Pharmaceutical Industry (1991)
Clinical Trial Compensation Guidelines. NHS bodies
are unable to offer indemnity in advance, but an
injured research subject would be able to pursue a
legal claim for negligence.

- Adequate information must be given to the prospec-
tive research subject to enable him or her to give valid
consent to participate in the research, and appropriate
procedures must be used to obtain and record that
consent. Particular care must be taken with those
research subjects who may be especially vulnerable,
e.g. children and the elderly. (Patient information
sheets and the consent process will be discussed more
fully later in this chapter.)

- Where a drug is to be used, the regulatory status of
that drug must be stated, and the proposals for its use
must be in accordance with what has been assented to
by the Medicines Control Agency.

- Where radioactive substances are to be used, the
investigator must hold a licence granted by the
Administration of Radioactive Substances Advisory
Committee (ARSAC).

- Any payments to a research subject must not be such
as to influence the subject's decision to participate in
the research. There is, at present, concern that
women may volunteer to have abortions, from which
fetal material can be used for research, to earn money.
Payments to research subjects must not be such as to
induce them to participate for reasons of monetary
gain, to the detriment of their own personal health.

- Where a research project is to be sponsored by an
outside organisation, any payments to the researcher
should be such that they do not call into question
the ethics of the research. For example, such payments should not constitute an inducement to the

researcher to continue to give a study drug beyond what is clinically indicated for the individual patient. Nurses with an involvement in studies being sponsored by commercial companies should bear such considerations in mind.

• It is necessary and appropriate to include the type of research subject that it is proposed to recruit (particular attention being paid to the inclusion of vulnerable groups, e.g. children).

• The nature of the research, i.e. therapeutic or non-therapeutic, should be clear.

• The research must be carried out in accordance with any EU Directives that may be applicable.

Special Groups

The involvement of certain groups of people in clinical research will be subject to particular scrutiny by an REC, and different and more stringent requirements may have to be met as a consequence of their participation. Such groups include children, healthy (non-patient) volunteers, pregnant and nursing women, women of childbearing age, the mentally disordered and prisoners.

Research involving children

The RCP guidelines (1990a) state that:

Children should not be the subject of research that might equally well be carried out on adults

while the *Guidelines for the Ethical Conduct of Medical Research Involving Children* (British Paediatric Association 1992) state that:

When a choice of age groups is possible, older children should be involved in preference to younger ones, although much valuable research can only be done with younger children and babies.

In assessing the risks of a research project to children who may be asked to participate, it is important to be aware of the special fears of children and that their reactions and responses will vary considerably, changing as they develop.

The question of consent to research on children is a complex one, and an REC will consider carefully how this is to be obtained in any project involving children as research subjects.

Research involving healthy (non-patient) volunteers

An REC will have particular requirements with regard to research involving healthy (non-patient) volunteers. Guidelines on *Research on Healthy Volunteers* have been produced by the RCP (1986).

Pregnant and nursing women and women of childbearing age

The restrictions on research involving pregnant and nursing women are discussed in paragraphs 13.5 and 13.6 of the RCP guidelines (1990a). In contemplating research on women of childbearing age, the possibility that they are or may become pregnant must be taken into consideration, and there must be good justification for their inclusion in the research.

Research involving the mentally disordered

There are special considerations in involving the mentally disorded in clinical research. *Guidelines for the Ethics of Research Committees on Psychiatric Research Involving Human*

Subjects have been produced by the Royal College of Psychiatrists (1989). Research involving the mentally disordered is also discussed in *Research Involving Patients* (RCP 1990b) and in *Guidelines on the Practice of Ethics Committees in Medical Research Involving Human Subjects* (RCP 1990a).

Research involving prisoners

Research involving prisoners is discussed in *Research Involving Patients* (RCP 1990b).

Research involving the use of fetuses and fetal material

A 'Code of Practice on the Use of Fetuses and Fetal Material in Research and Treatment' is to be found in Appendix B of the DoH guidelines (1991). This has been taken from the Polkinghorne Report, *Review of the Guidance on the Research Use of Fetuses and Fetal Material* (1989).

Multicentre Research

If the research project is being undertaken in more than one institution, applicants should be aware that the REC in each participating centre has the right to review and give or withhold ethical approval of the work being undertaken in that institution. At the very least, this may be irritating and frustrating for researchers, particularly where different committees may express differing or even contrary views about the same project. At the very worst, it may be argued that life-saving research could be impeded or prevented from taking place. Although in its guidelines (1991) the DoH states that:

> committees should arrive at a voluntary arrangement under which one LREC is nominated to consider the issue on behalf of them all

and goes on to say that:

> Health Authorities should positively encourage networks
> for neighbouring LRECs so that such co-operation is
> more easily achieved.

This is more easily said than done, and the DoH offers no advice as to how this might be achieved. On a practical level, much collaboration in research does not take place in 'neighbouring' institutions but across district, national and international boundaries. It is also possible that many RECs and the bodies that constitute them would be reluctant to give up their independence and right to review all research that will take place in that institution.

As standards of ethical review improve, it is likely that RECs will become more consistent but also more stringent in their requirements. While increased consistency should foster trust and cooperation between committees and facilitate cooperation in the ethical review process, increased stringency and the introduction of the internal market in the health service may serve to make RECs, and the institutions which constitute them and give permission for studies to go ahead, more reluctant to accept decisions taken elsewhere.

The question of how best to deal with the ethical review of multicentre research is currently the subject of much debate, and as yet there is no agreed solution.

The Patient Information Sheet

For the vast majority of research studies, the REC will require that a patient information sheet be prepared and made available to all potential research subjects. Exception to this might be made only in circumstances in which there was considered to be no risk and minimal inconvenience to the research subject.

The patient information sheet is intended to be a summary of the information the potential research subject needs to know in order to make a valid decision as to whether or not to participate in the proposed research. It should not be regarded by the researcher as a substitute for verbal communication but as a supportive document to reinforce the information given verbally. The patient information sheet should be given to the potential research subject to keep and use as an aide-mémoire, both while making a decision as to whether or not to participate and, if agreeing to participate, during the course of the study.

The patient information sheet should be clear and concise and preferably contained within one or two sides of a sheet of paper. It should be worded as an 'invitation' to participate in the proposed research and should make it clear, from the outset, that what is proposed is research rather than standard treatment. The use of medical jargon should be avoided, and essential medical terminology should be explained so that the information can easily be understood by the potential research subject.

The RCP guidelines *Research Involving Patients* (1990b) state that 'The Information Sheet should be separate from the Consent Form'. There are, however, arguments in favour of the two documents being combined. It would seem reasonable that the research subject should not only be able to retain the written information given to him or her about a research study but also be able to retain a copy of any document that has been signed. One combined copy, rather than two separate documents, might be more convenient for the research subject to keep, the top copy of the document being retained by the researcher. This could also have the advantage of facilitating any monitoring of the consent and information process.

The content of the patient information sheet will vary according to the nature of the study proposed, but the

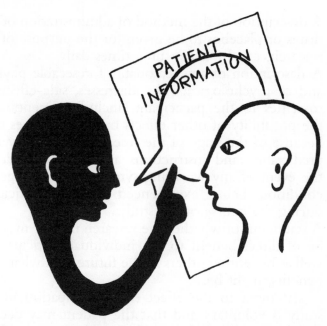

following is offered as a list of elements that should be considered for inclusion.

- An explanation of the nature and purpose of the research, including the methodology of the study, e.g. involving randomisation or use of a placebo.
- Details of the expected duration of the research subject's overall participation: for example, the number and duration of out-patient appointments, investigations or in-patient stays; the anticipated time it will take to complete or undergo a questionnaire or interview; and the time-span covered by the study, including any period of follow-up.
- A description (including any resulting discomforts) of any procedures or investigations to be undertaken for the purposes of the study, e.g. venepuncture, x-rays or scans (highlighting any that may be experimental).

- A description of the method of administration of any drugs or placebos to be given for the purpose of the research, e.g. by tablet three times daily.
- A description of any reasonably foreseeable physical and/or psychological risks, distresses, side-effects or toxicities to the participant, including mention of the possibility of other effects or consequences that, because of the stage of the research, may not yet be predictable, and instructions as to what to do in the event of any worrying symptoms or changes in condition being experienced by the participant during the course of the study.
- A statement of whether the research may or may not be of direct benefit to the individual participant as well as benefiting others in the future, and what such benefits might be.
- A statement to the effect that participation in the study is voluntary and that the patient may decline to take part or withdraw during the course of the research, his or her decision being accepted without having to give a reason and without recrimination or disadvantage to his or her future care.
- A statement to the effect that the researcher may consider it in the participant's best interests to withdraw him or her from the study and offer an alternative treatment or methods of care.
- A description of the steps that will be taken to maintain confidentiality with respect to individual participants, including mention of any possibility that medical records will be inspected and by whom.
- A statement to the effect that the participant's legal rights will not be affected by giving consent to take part in the study.
- An explanation of any arrangements that may have been made (by any non-NHS body collaborating in the study) for compensating the participant in the

event of any injury to him or her arising out of the project.

- The name, work address and telephone number of at least one researcher involved in the study whom the participant may contact, particularly if he or she is worried about any change in health during the course of the study or if he or she has any queries about the project, either before, during or after participation.

- A statement to the effect tht the participant is entitled to be informed about the results or findings of the study if he or she so wishes, and how and when this information will be made available.

- An explanation of the existence or otherwise of any other forms of treatment or care that may be available as an alternative to participation in the research.

- A statement to the effect that the research subject's general practitioner will be notified of his or her participation in the study (if this is appropriate to the nature of the research).

- A statement to the effect that the research project has been approved by an REC, that the participant has the right of access to the REC if he or she has concerns about the research or participation in it that have not been resolved by discussion with the researcher, and how such access may be gained.

The inclusion in the patient information sheet of a statement such as that suggested in the last item above will, at the time of writing, be considered by some to be controversial, and it would be interesting to know how many RECs make this a requirement.

The question of how such an item should be worded is left open but should be the subject of careful consideration. It would be important to ensure that a statement to the effect that a study had been approved by an REC did not have the effect of exerting undue pressure to participate and creating a perception that, because the REC had approved a study, participation was especially recommended or that there would be no possible risks in participation.

In informing the research subject of his or her right of access to the REC, it would be important to ensure that, in order to avoid compromising the relationship between the researcher (who may also be the person responsible for the overall care of the research subject) and the research subject, such access was reserved for raising matters of serious concern not resolved by discussion with the researcher and should not be seen by the research subject as an alternative means of obtaining information, advice or reassurance that could more appropriately be given by the researcher.

Consent To Participate in Clinical Research

Obtaining consent to participate in clinical research is central to the ethical conduct of a research study, and how this will be obtained and recorded will be of particular interest and concern to an REC in considering an application for ethical approval of a research project. It is particularly important, therefore, to ensure that the way in which it is proposed to go about this has been well thought through and is appropriate to the nature of the intended research.

In general, no clinical research may be conducted on a subject unless he or she is aware that what is proposed is research and has been given sufficient information, in a form which is understandable, to enable him or her to make an independent and considered decision to agree to participate in the research. Such 'valid' consent must be given and recorded either orally or in writing. However, the RCP suggests in its guidelines (1990a) and in *Research Involving Patients* (1990b) that there may be some circumstances in which an REC may agree to research being carried out without the consent of the subject. These include:

- observational research involving no risk to or participation of the research subject, an example being given as 'a study involving the measurement of the amount of food not eaten by patients and its relationship to the spontaneously occurring variation in delay in serving meals';
- research into comprehension or behaviour, where the results of the study would be compromised by the research subject's awareness of the matter under scrutiny. This may only be permitted if the research carries no more than minimal risk, if the prior approval of an REC is sought and if the subject is subsequently informed that the observations have been made and gives 'deferred consent';
- some unintrusive community research (provided that confidentiality is preserved);
- examination of anonymous specimens provided during the course of routine medical practice, no longer required for that purpose and which would otherwise be discarded, the use of remnants of specimens previously provided for clincial purposes and the use for related research purposes of stored specimens previously provided for research into the disease from which the patient suffered;
- minor procedures involving minimal risk and no or negligible discomfort to the research subject, and where it is considered that to seek consent would be more likely to cause distress than to proceed without it. In such instances, it is proposed that the procedures involved should cause no more discomfort than that

normally experienced by a patient undergoing diagnostic tests as part of routine care. Examples given are 'collection of urine and faeces, nasal and throat swabs and the withdrawal of a small extra volume of blood while blood is being taken for a necessary diagnostic process';

- major procedures or urgent situations, such as when a patient has a rare, severe or not well understood condition, when it would be 'impossible or devastating' to attempt to obtain consent, e.g. following trauma, sudden cardiac arrest, when comprehension is impaired and where research into the management of the illness or condition is proposed, provided that the research subject is subsequently informed of what has taken place and 'deferred consent' is obtained, if appropriate. Where research continues after the 'unexpected initiating event', prior consent to continued participation should be sought;
- research involving only access to personal medical records as a source of information, providing that scrupulous care is taken to ensure patient confidentiality. In all cases in which it is not proposed to seek the prior consent of the research subject to participate in a clinical research project, the REC should be consulted in advance and its approval obtained.

Mode of Consent to Research

Consent to participate in clinical research may be given orally or in writing. Rarely, the fact of a research subject undertaking what is required of him or her as a consequence of participating in a study, for example completion of a questionnaire, may be taken as evidence of consent having been given. However, this would only be appropriate in research of an innocuous nature.

The difference between these two modes of consent rests largely on the way in which the consent of the research subject is recorded, although it may be acceptable, depending upon the nature of the study proposed, for oral consent to be accompanied by only an oral explanation of the research, whereas written consent should always be sought only after both oral and written explanations of the research have been given.

In oral consent, the person seeking consent and an independent witness to the consent process are required to record in writing that sufficient information has been given for the potential research subject to give valid consent and that he or she has had the opportunity to ask questions, has understood the purpose and nature of what is proposed, is satisfied with the information that has been given and has consented to participate voluntarily.

In written consent, the potential research subject, together with the person seeking consent and an independent witness to the consent process, is required to record in writing on a consent form the same elements as those listed above for oral consent, with the potential research subject signing a statement to the effect that he or she agrees to participate.

In its guidelines (1990a), the RCP advises that:

> Research Ethics Committees should exercise discretion as to the mode of consent that is appropriate to the nature of the proposed research.

There are no hard and fast rules, but this is generally taken to mean that the more invasive or intrusive the research and the greater the risk, the more stringent the requirements with regard to consent will be. Because there are no exact rules or one preferred mode of consent for all research, the requirements of different RECs will vary. Consent procedures are the subject of much discussion, and, of late, requirements have become much more stringent, with the development of a trend towards seeking signed rather than oral consent. In fact, the DoH guidelines *Local Research Ethics Committees* (1991) propose that:

Written consent should be required for all research (except where the most trivial of procedures is concerned).

Oral consent may still be considered appropriate in the case of research which is easy for the potential research subject to understand and where less than minimal risk is involved. Examples of this might be a questionnaire about diet or measurement of height and weight. Oral consent may have the advantage of being less intimidating for the potential research subject.

In both its guidelines (1990a) and *Research Involving Patients* (1990b), the RCP suggests that witnessed (oral) consent is 'especially useful in the old and in those who have intellectual or cultural difficulties in speech or understanding, or who are distressed, but who are deemed capable of giving consent'. However, it could be argued that, both ethically and practically, the advisability of seeking to recruit such groups of patients is doubtful, that special care should be taken in consenting them and that, by virtue of the difficulties that such potential research subjects are experiencing, verbal consent is inappropriate. A disadvantage of oral consent is that it may not, to the same extent as written consent, serve to highlight that what is proposed is research rather than standard treatment.

Written or signed consent has, in the past, been considered to be more intimidating than oral consent. This argument is perhaps less relevant now that patients are required to give written consent to all routine treatments or investigations that carry any substantial risks or side effects and will, therefore, have the opportunity to become more familiar with the requirement to give written consent. In the same way, the argument that written consent serves to highlight that what is being proposed is research rather than routine treatment becomes less valid.

A disadvantage of written consent might be that, in the event of a dispute between the researcher and the research subject, the consent document may be used to protect the researcher rather than the person it was designed to protect — the research subject. However, this could also be said of any document recording oral consent.

It should be noted that opinions vary on the value of obtaining the research subject's signature on a consent form. In its guidelines (1990a), the RCP states that it is likely that:

> a court of law would look at any such document in the context of the whole investigation and might at best regard it as evidence that the investigator has seriously endeavoured to meet his responsibilities.

Certainly, by giving written consent, the research subject in no way loses his or her statutory rights to take legal action in the event of any concern arising out of his or her participation in a research study, nor does it absolve the researcher from any of his or her responsibilities.

However, an important advantage of written consent is that a well-designed consent document may be used by the potential research subject, the person seeking consent and the independent witness as a 'checklist' for ensuring that all elements of the consent process have been adhered to. An example of such a document is put forward by the RCP in *Research Involving Patients* (1990b), although this makes no provision for signature by only the research subject.

Seeking and Gaining Consent

It is not the fact of obtaining consent, whether oral or written, that is important, but rather the way in which
— this is achieved. Consent freely given but based on a lack of understanding or inadequate information would be worthless, as would consent given as a result of coercion.

In general, the person seeking consent will be a member of the research team, although Palmer (1991) suggests that, in order to avoid any question of duress or coercion arising, the person seeking consent should be someone not connected with the research project. Whoever the person seeking consent may be, it is important that he or she has a thorough knowledge of what is proposed, can communicate well and is able to answer any questions that may be asked about the research by the potential research subject.

The purpose of having an independent witness to the consent process is to protect the interests of the potential research subject. Most commonly, the witness will be a nurse or other member of hospital staff but, in theory, could be anyone chosen by the potential research subject. It can be argued that, since it is a nurse's role to protect a patient's interests, it is entirely appropriate that she or he should act in the capacity of independent witness and, by virtue of her or his knowledge and experience, be well placed to:

- understand what is proposed;
- assist the potential research subject to understand what is proposed;
- have an awareness of the quantity and quality of information that has been given;
- judge whether any consent given is 'valid'.

Equally well, it could be said that a nurse or other member of hospital staff, particularly if the person is a member of the research team, could have an interest in or be under pressure to recruit research subjects to a study and, fore, cannot be truly 'independent'.

The exact procedure to be adopted when seeking consent will vary according to the nature of the research. In general, the first step should be to give a full verbal explanation of the research, together with the patient information sheet. The person who is seeking consent or acting as a witness may find it helpful to go through the information sheet with the potential research subject, using this document as an aide-mémoire and checklist to ensure that all the necessary points have been covered. Rarely, it may be appropriate (with the prior approval of the REC) to dispense with either the verbal or written explanation.

In all cases, the potential recruit must be given time to consider the proposal. In general, the more complicated the research and the more significant the risks or implications of participation, the more time should be given for reflection. There will be few situations in which it will be appropriate to seek and require consent to be given on the same day, exceptions being situations of extreme urgency or research of an unintrusive nature bearing no risk.

The potential research subject should be able to take away with him or her the patient information sheet and discuss the proposal with anyone of his or her choosing. Where written consent is being sought and the consent form and patient information sheet are separate, a copy of the consent form may also be offered, so that the potential recruit will have time to read what he or she will be asked to sign. However, it should be made clear that the form should not be signed unless in the presence of the person seeking consent and the witness. Opportunities should be given for the potential recruit to ask questions, not only when first being informed about the research, but also during the period of reflection and, later, when consent is sought.

If necessary, and particularly when the research is complicated and/or the potential recruit may also have had to take in complicated and/or distressing information about his or her medical condition, the explanation of the research should be repeated on more than one occasion. The person responsible for seeking consent or acting as an independent witness may find it helpful to ask the potential recruit what he or she thinks is the nature and purpose of the research and his or her participation in it. The witness to the consent procedure should not sign the form unless satisfied that the consent being given is 'valid'.

Finally, once completed, all forms recording both oral and written consent should be filed in a patient's medical records or, in the case of non-patient volunteers, kept carefully with the study records. Any other requirements of the REC with regard to the retention and storage of completed consent forms should be complied with.

Responsibilities of the Investigator whose Project has Received Ethical Approval

Once the project has been submitted and has received ethical approval, the applicant should ensure that, in conducting the study, any specific conditions that have been laid down by the REC, upon which ethical approval is conditional, have been met. In particular, it is important to adhere to any conditions laid down with regard to informing, consenting and maintaining the confidentiality of the potential research subjects.

All those concerned with the care of the research subjects participating in the project must be aware of the study and a copy of the protocol made available to them. Reports on the progress of the study must be submitted to the REC upon request, and any adverse or unforeseen events arising out of the project must be immediately

reported to the committee. Should it become n
during the course of the study, to make any sig
changes to the project, the prior approval of th̲ ҡЕС
must be sought. Failure to meet the requirements of the
REC in any way could result in ethical approval being
withdrawn.

Confidentiality

A key responsibility of a researcher, both during and after
the completion of a study, is to ensure that the confidentiality of the research subject is preserved, and the REC
will be concerned that due care and attention is paid to
ensuring this.

The UKCC *Code of Professional Conduct* (1992) states
that registered nurses, midwives and health visitors must:

> protect all confidential information concerning patients and
> clients obtained in the course of professional practice
> and make disclosures only with consent.

Nurses must be aware of their responsibilities with regard
to maintaining the confidentiality of research subjects,
whether they are the investigator or are assisting in the
conduct of a study during the course of their daily work.

All information gained about a research subject during
the course of his or her participation in the research must
be treated as confidential. This applies equally to information volunteered by the research subject, for example
in response to a questionnaire, and to data obtained from
medical records during the course of a retrospective case
note review.

As a general rule, the more sensitive the information
obtained, the more care must be taken to preserve confidentiality. Ideally, and provided that safety is in no way
compromised, any specimens collected for the purpose

of a research study, or any questionnaires or data sheets completed, should be coded rather than bear the name (or any other information from which an individual might be identified) of the research subject. This is particularly important where specimens or data are being sent for analysis outside the organisation.

Care must be taken to ensure that all data or specimens collected for the purposes of a research study are stored securely. Special considerations will apply to personal data stored on computer, and researchers should be aware of the requirements of the Data Protection Act (1984).

Where studies are being undertaken in collaboration with a commercial company, it may sometimes be necessary for audit purposes for an official of the company to inspect the original medical records of the research subject. This is permissible, but the records must be viewed within the organisation legally responsible for them, and the research subject should be informed that this will be necessary before he or she gives consent to participate in the research.

In publishing the results of the research, the confidentiality of the research subject must be preserved. In some studies of a qualitative nature involving a small number of research subjects, this may, in some cases, actually prove quite difficult. Such studies are often undertaken by nurses, and they must take particular care when presenting or publishing the results.

More detailed and general advice may be found in the UKCC Advisory Paper *Confidentiality* (1987).

Conclusion

As society changes and medicine and technology advance, new ethical issues relating to research on human beings will arise. In the course of their work, and as members of society who may themselves be potential research subjects, nurses have a duty not only to be aware of existing ethical debates and requirements relating to research, but also to keep abreast of new ethical issues and the work and requirements of RECs. They also have a duty to make their views known and participate in the ongoing process of formulating ethical guidelines and upholding the principles of good ethical practice in research.

References

Association of the British Pharmaceutical Industry (1991) *Clinical Trial Compensation Guidelines*. London: The Association of the British Pharmaceutical Industry.

British Paediatric Association (1992) *Guidelines for the Ethical Conduct of Medical Research Involving Children*. London: British Paediatric Association.

Campbell A V (1989) Power and responsibility in the practice of medicine. *Studies in Christian Ethics*, 2 (1): pp. 5–16.

Data Protection Act (1984) London: HMSO.

Department of Health (1991) Health Service Guidelines HSG(91)5 *Local Research Ethics Committees*. London: Department of Health.

Hunt G (1992) Nursing and ethics committees. *Ethics Forum Issue 4*. London: National Centre for Nursing and Midwifery Ethics, Queen Charlotte's College.

Neuberger J (1992) *Ethics and Health Care: The Role of Research Ethics Committees in the United Kingdom*. Research Report 13. London: King's Fund Institute.

Palmer R N (1991) Consent and Confidentiality. In J P Jackson (ed.) *A Practical Guide to Medicine and the Law*. London: Springer-Verlag.

Polkinghorne Report (1989) *Review of the Guidance on the Research Use of Fetuses and Fetal Material*. Cmnd 762. London: HMSO.

Royal College of Physicians (1986) *Research on Healthy Volunteers*. London: RCP.

Royal College of Physicians (1990a) *Guidelines on the Practice of Ethics Committees in Medical Research Involving Human Subjects* (2nd edn.). London: RCP.

Royal College of Physicians (1990b) *Research Involving Patients.* London: RCP.

Royal College of Psychiatrists (1989) *Guidelines for the Ethics of Research Committees on Psychiatric Research Involving Human Subjects.* London: Royal College of Psychiatrists.

UKCC (1987) *Confidentiality. An elaboration of Clause 9 of the Second Edition of the UKCC's Code of Professional Conduct for the Nurse, Midwife and Health Visitor.* London: UKCC.

UKCC (1992) *Code of Professional Conduct for the Nurse, Midwife and Health Visitor* (3rd edn.). London: UKCC.

World Medical Association Declaration of Helsinki (1964; amended Tokyo 1975, Venice 1983 and Hong Kong 1989) *Recommendations Guiding Physicians in Biomedical Research Involving Human Subjects.* New York: World Medical Association.

Further Reading

Centre of Medical Law and Ethics (1992) *Manual for Research Ethics Committees.* Compiled by Claire Gilbert Foster. London: Centre of Medical Law and Ethics, King's College. The *Manual for Research Ethics Committees* is essential reading for any nurse appointed to serve as a member of an REC. It is also an excellent source of information with respect to research ethics requirements. It contains a number of the guidelines referred to in this chapter.

European Commission (1991) Directive of 19 July 1991 modifying the Annex to Council Directive 75/318/EEC on the approximation of the laws of Member States relating to analytical, pharmacotoxological and clinical standards and protocols in respect of the testing of medicinal products (91/507/EEC). *Official Journal of the European Communities*, 26.9.91, no. L 270/32.

CHAPTER 4

Sponsorship

Gillian Little

Ethics in health care happens mostly on the borderline between the known and acceptable and the not yet fully known and, therefore, not yet quite acceptable. Commercial sponsorship of nursing posts is one of these grey areas.

The author, who writes from a perspective of clinical nurse specialist in stoma care, gives the reader an overview of the many issues involved in sponsorship, and its gains and risks, and also poses some questions that may have to be asked more specifically in the future if this form of providing health care is here to stay.

Is sponsorship in nursing here to stay? What precisely does the term 'sponsorship' mean anyway, and does it have any implications for nursing practice?

A possible scenario is a hospital surgical department that is about to lose one of its specialist nursing posts due to chronic overspending. A company contacts the hospital manager and offers to fund the post. The nurse works within the agreement drawn up between hospital manager and company manager, and the specialist nursing post is protected.

But is this all there is to sponsorship — a mutually beneficial deal whereby all parties gain something? (The patient is generally a third party in the deal, somewhere in the middle.) If this is all there is, nurses as primary patient carers have little, if anything, to concern themselves with.

Before we can be comfortable with this conclusion, however, we need to consider what a sponsorship agree-

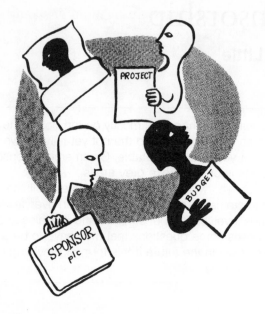

ment entails and whether or not there is any ethical dilemma for the nurse involved.

Nurses joining the profession today find themselves entering the arena at a time when many fundamental shifts in the way that nursing care is delivered are taking place. In many instances, some form of sponsorship will form an integral part of the delivery of health care within the nurse's workplace, health authority or trust. Whether or not there is an issue to consider regarding the ethics of sponsorship depends to a large extent on the capacity within such an agreement for the independence of the nurse's judgement. This is borne out by the UKCC *Code of Professional Conduct* (1992), clause 16, which states that:

> As a registered nurse, midwife or health visitor, you are personally accountable for your practice and, in the exercise of your professional accountability, must . . . ensure that your registration status is not used in the promotion of commercial products or services, declare any financial or

other interests in relevant organisations providing such goods or services and ensure that your professional judgement is not influenced by any commercial considerations.

Many nurses have an intuitive grasp of what is right and wrong for their patients, which reflects the theory that ethics is not necessarily derived from experience or logic, but rather from intuition, humans automatically or instinctively possessing an understanding of right and wrong.

Sponsorship: Some Facts

A common form of sponsorship is that of indirect sponsorship from a disinterested party (although this has little relevance to the issues of concern explored in this chapter). An example of this is a company making spare parts for motor vehicles, which may find it beneficial to sponsor its local hospital Accident and Emergency department, which is in turn fundraising for waiting room facilities. In return for an agreed amount per annum, the company may secure advertising space at an agreed location within the department. The department is able to purchase the much-needed equipment sooner, and the sponsoring company benefits locally from its advertised association with a caring environment. There is no involvement with or relationship to the delivery of clinical practice. The sponsoring company has no specific interest in the business of the Accident and Emergency department, other than that of its providing a suitable medium for the advertisement.

More direct forms of sponsorship usually involve specialist nursing posts and companies who have a direct interest in the specialty concerned, e.g. stoma care. The fact that it is highly profitable for some companies to offer a considerable level of sponsored funding can be borne out by the historical fact that the sponsorship of such posts has been offered to hospital managers who had no declared need for a service to be 'rescued'.

The nurse working in a directly sponsored post will generally be required to stock and use the sponsoring company's product or service and provide an agreed level of information regarding product usage figures (including competitors' product usage) to the sponsor on a regular basis.

It is assumed that those considering sponsorship of nursing services for the first time will pay close attention to the more obvious areas of the nurse's freedom of judgement and facilitation of unbiased patient choice of appliances, believing that these are the only issues to be addressed. However, this is often not so. Companies known to be involved in offering sponsorship to fund or support posts in stoma care nursing all hold product dispensing licences, which means that they are in the business of dispensing prescriptions of ostomy equipment to those patients who send in their prescriptions. Any company's equipment can be stored for dispensing; the profit lies in the highly complex reimbursement schemes for prescription items applicable within the UK at the present time. In other words, for the sponsoring company it is more profitable to dispense prescriptions to a stoma patient than to rely solely on its products being recommended in sufficient quantities to the patient in hospital. This can be borne out by the fact that a sponsorship agreement of the type described, i.e. an amount equivalent to the nurse's annual salary, has, in the main, only been offered where part of the agreement involves the nurse's promotion of the company's prescription dispensing service when the patient has a stated preference not to use his or her local chemist.

The stoma patient is likely to represent a long-term level of income via prescription reimbursement for the sponsoring company because most patients tend to obtain a prescription for bags and accessories every month. If the patient is using a type of bag manufactured by the sponsor, the level of potential profit will be even greater.

Ostomy Appliance Prescription Dispensing

All retail pharmacists (chemists) will dispense prescriptions for ostomy appliances. Some pharmacists go to great lengths to assist their customers by offering home delivery. There are also a number of dispensing appliance contractors whose sole business is the receiving and dispensing of ostomy appliance prescriptions. There are also some ostomy appliance manufacturers who have made dispensing an additional business. The level of patient service is generally greater than that received via a chemist. Free disposal bags and tissue cleansers, a free appliance aperture cutting service and a freephone advice line will accompany the actual dispensing of bags. The two-pronged effect of potential profit for the manufacturer who also dispenses is thus evident.

Could a nurse be placed in an ethically compromising situation from involvement with such a sponsoring arrangement? Nurses are aware that they must be seen to work in accordance with the UKCC *Code of Professional Conduct* (1992). There are also issues of patient advocacy and nurse impartiality when functioning in a specialist capacity in which several commercial organisations have equal interest. Is there, then, potential for coercion? There may well be a level of anxiety of possible withdrawal of sponsor funding if the sponsor does not feel that he is seeing sufficient return against investment.

These possible conflicts of interest bear further investigation. In the light of the development of hospital trusts and the effects of the internal market upon us all, can this type of sponsorship be due purely to retailing change or is something more insidious going on?

Why Sponsor — Issues of Gain

Gain is here examined from the perspectives of each party involved:

- The hospital manager.
- The patient.
- The nurse.
- The sponsoring product manufacturer.

The hospital manager

The subject of nursing ethics will have no place on the hospital manager's agenda. It is sufficient for him or her to ensure that any agreement with a sponsor falls within the scope of the law, is workable and is profitable for the hospital. He or she will also wish to ensure that any outcomes from an agreement of this kind between industry and health care can be seen to be in the best interest of the patients, not necessarily just those whom it will affect. Therefore, the hospital manager's gain will arise from:

- the provision of a service, if one did not exist prior to the sponsorship agreement;
- the extension of a service, were its continuation threatened due to lack of funds;
- income generation to the health authority or trust, to the tune of around £19,000 (G and H grade salaries, 1994 figures).

The patient

Patients in the throes of a major illness will find themselves at an extremely vulnerable point in their lives. Psychologically, coping mechanisms and decision-making abilities will often desert them with devastating speed, exposing them to raw dependence on the knowledge and guidance of the medical profession. As Kelly (1985) wrote:

> Once I had come to terms with my newly acquired patient status . . . I placed absolute trust, not to say faith, in the technical competence of the professionals. Any doubt I may have entertained about the staff's ability was, for my part, repressed as I suspended disbelief for the duration of my stay.

In Orem's (1985) theory of nursing, the relevance of these comments can be reinforced by looking at the three systems of nursing described, which all consider self-care, in both the physical and emotional sense, to be the crux of nursing:

- *The wholly compensatory system* — which is needed when the patient's capacity for self-care is temporarily or permanently destroyed. In such situations, caring is manifested through acting for and doing for the patient.
- *The partly compensatory system* — which is used when patients can help themselves a little. The caring act is demonstrated by doing for patients and helping them to do for themselves.
- *The supportive-educative system* — which is used for those patients who need only support and guidance. Caring, here, lies in the encouragement of the patient's own autonomy.

Accepting that the patient will have a varying need for caring intervention, the issue of gain for the patient is dependent upon having access to carers who are suitably qualified to be able to recognise and meet specific needs. Therefore, if a clinical nurse specialist has become available to that patient as a result of a sponsorship agreement rendering this service viable, it can be suggested that a positive contribution to the patient's eventual rehabilitation has been received. However, taken in isolation, this viewpoint could be said to be rather altruistic, and in order to be able to formulate an objective appraisal, one has to consider the nurse's role specifically in terms of her or his impartiality while working within such an agreement, and being an advocate for the patient, before evaluating the net benefit to the patient.

The nurse

Any gain for a nurse is obviously going to be dependent on the reasoning behind the sponsorship agreement and whether or not the nurse was privy to the compilation of the agreement.

If the job of an existing stoma care nurse is under threat due to lack of hospital funds and a sponsorship deal allows that service to continue, or if a ward sister who wishes to specialise is only able to do so with the funding of a commercial sponsor, an immediate gain becomes apparent. It must also be remembered that with sponsorship by an interested party, the very existence of the role is totally due to the sponsor's input.

The whole ethos of any sponsorship agreement is that it should be mutually beneficial, and within stoma care nursing, the contact between sponsor and nurse is frequent, while the contact between sponsor and hospital management is sporadic. Therefore, the nurse will have constant reinforcement that she or he functions under the terms of a sponsorship agreement, by agreeing to provide the sponsor with regular (usually monthly) information. In stoma care, this relates specifically to new stoma surgery statistical information and the appliance type selected and used on discharge. Within this environment, the nurse has constantly to be aware of and functioning within the scope of the UKCC *Code of Professional Conduct*. In April 1990, the UKCC issued a statement on commercial sponsorship and the position of nurses, midwives and health visitors, which states that:

> the Council recognises that proposals for funding some posts, projects and specific services may increasingly come from commercial sources. The same principles set out in relation to advertising apply, that is independence of professional judgement based on the needs of the patients and clients, unfettered by undue commercial influence.

The sponsoring product manufacturer

Under the terms of the sponsoring agreement, the manufacturer's products will be offered to every patient, as appropriate. For example, the colostomy bag range will be offered to every patient with a colostomy who is seen by the nurse. In some agreements, the sponsor requests that their bag be the one used as first choice. Either way, there is an increased chance of the sponsor's products being used, which will result in increased sales for the company. If the patient cannot or does not wish to use the sponsor's product, there is still a chance for further gain via the use of the sponsor's prescription service on the patient's discharge home. (Manufacturers offering a prescription service will stock any other manufacturer's bags, ready for dispensing when patients send in their prescription.)

Considering that the average in-patient stay for ostomy surgery is 14–21 days, there is a natural limit to the number of bags that can be used by a patient in that time. It is the amount of business available after discharge that is of greater value to any sponsor, particularly with ostomy patients, as this is often a lifetime requirement. Evidence has shown that the bag type that a patient selects for use while in hospital is often used continually thereafter, although alternative choice is extensive and samples are readily available if desired. This situation may help to explain why a majority of the sponsoring offers made to date have been towards hospital-based stoma care services. Indeed, one community-based stoma care nurse informed the Stoma Care Nurses Forum that her sponsors had withdrawn funding due to the lack of their product being used.

Therefore, the sponsor can gain either by the increased uptake of their manufactured products or by the patients' use of their prescription service. If there is no gain for the product manufacturer, funding may be withdrawn.

Is There a Risk of Coercion?

What of the nurse who holds her or his position as special-ist nurse solely because of the commercial sponsor? If the position of an employee relies solely on continued funding from a sponsor, this is not such a problem if the sponsor is a disinterested party who has no say in day-to-day clinical decisions and whose objectives do not rely on patient outcomes.

Is there a problem for a nurse in this situation with an ostomy product manufacturer as the sponsor? There appears to be a balancing act of sorts going on here. Nurses will certainly be aware of their obligations towards the UKCC *Code of Professional Conduct*. Also, if there is insuf-ficient use of the commercial sponsor's product or service, funding is in danger of being withdrawn. What con-clusions must nurses now come to with regard to their obligations to the sponsor? (Some health service employers have agreed to accept the ongoing funding of the role if a sponsor withdraws funding for any reason. In these

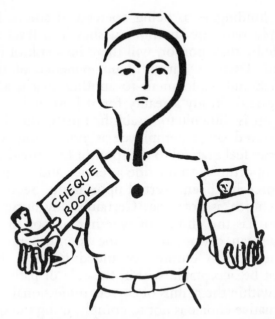

circumstances, there is a safety margin for nurses to exercise their professional judgement with a degree of freedom. However, for other health authorities, this is not an option that has been built in to the sponsorship agreement. If the sponsor withdraws funding, the service is discontinued, with resultant loss to both the patients who had enjoyed access to that service and the nurse who may no longer be able to work within that specialty.)

Coercion, basically, means lack of choice, being unable to refuse an unfair bargain. The most obvious cases in business would be those in which employees are forced to take an unpleasant or dangerous job rather than be fired or demoted. This has been described as the opposite of freedom as well as the instrument of injustice (Solomon and Hanson, 1983). It could be said that the nurse who is a party to the worst example of sponsorship — interested party with no commitment on the part of the employer to continue funding in the event of withdrawal of the sponsor's funding — is being coerced. If she or he does not comply with the sponsor's wishes to a level deemed acceptable by that sponsor, will there be a risk of firing or demotion? There is currently no evidence of this, but loss of post and deployment to another area is a distinct possibility, and already a reality for at least one nurse.

Coercion is difficult to establish. Firstly, the degree of 'force' exerted on an employee is not readily obvious. Some nurses feel grateful to the sponsor for providing them with an opportunity to provide a service and sincerely feel that no force has been exerted upon them. Secondly, the issue of 'choice' is not clear. Certainly, any nurse in such a situation has the choice of whether or not to comply. She or he can choose to use the sponsor's product or service heavily, to ensure continued funding, but this would not be acceptable within the role of patient advocate, nor within the realms of correct professional conduct. The alternative choice is not to comply, using the sponsor's products and service in equal amounts with those of its competitors, hoping that this will be enough to ensure continued funding.

This changes the question of whether the nurse has choice to whether there is an *acceptable* choice, which is altogether more difficult to consider. The issue of coercion strikes right at the heart of any discussion of economic rights and justice in a free enterprise system. The reverse of this argument is that as long as everyone else acts within their own rights, the employee who is forced to take an unsatisfactory role is not coerced. Necessity is not necessarily coercion. Is this the prudent stance we should be taking when considering service delivery in today's health care market?

The Nurse as Patient Advocate

The concept of the nurse as an advocate of the patient is one that appears with increasing frequency in the heightened politically aware culture of nursing in the 1990s. There are many definitions of the term 'advocate'. Among the more traditional (International Council of Nurses, 1973) is that:

> The nurse's primary commitment is to the patients' care and safety. She must be alert to take appropriate action regarding any instances of incompetence, unethical or illegal practice by any member of the health care team, or any action on the part of others that is prejudicial to the patients' best interests.

A rather less defensive stance is offered by Gadow (1980), who states that individuals 'should be assisted by nursing to authentically exercise their freedom and self-determination'.

The role that nurses will adopt in the fulfilment of their function as advocates is facilitated by the degree of freedom and autonomy employed in the exercise of nursing. Critics of sponsorship in nursing have frequently expressed concern that enforced allegiance to any single commercial agent, such as a sponsor who is allowed direct involvement in the delivery of nursing care (or decision-making, which is likely to affect nursing outcomes), will undermine this role by impinging upon the freedom of choice and autonomy with which a nurse can choose the most appropriate model of nursing care, aimed at promoting the patient's physical and psychological rehabilitation. A possible means of avoiding this perceived risk is to distance the sponsor from the nurse who is sponsored, that is, to ensure that contact between the two parties is handled by an intermediary, perhaps the hospital manager, who holds responsibility for arranging the working agreement at the outset.

If the sponsor originates from an unassociated industry, this issue ceases to be a risk as there is little gain in such an industry monitoring the nurse's decision-making and patient-care planning activities.

Whether there is a real threat to the nurse's role as advocate in the presence of a direct sponsor is for the reader to decide. It is, however, of vital importance that the existence of this function and its place in quality nursing care is truly valued and nurtured. As Witts (1992) stated:

> When we consider the notion of quality of patient care, we are of necessity committing ourselves to a discussion of ethics and moral values as they relate to both physical and psychological well-being. In this way advocacy can be seen to have profound consequences for the quality of psychology care.

Risk Control Systems

For hospital managers seeking income generation strategies to relieve some strain on already stretched budgets, both the short- and long-term outcomes of accepting the option of sponsorship need to be understood by and acceptable to the various parties involved. Whether a direct or indirect sponsor should be selected may be the first decision to be made. If it is a nursing post to be sponsored, would it be pertinent to consider some risk control systems at this stage, being aware that any commercial sponsor's interest is unlikely to be completely altruistic?

Johnson and Scholes (1989) make the point that:

> The likely return from a particular strategy is an important measure of the acceptability of that strategy. However, there is another, different, measure of acceptability against which strategic options might need to be assessed. This is the *risk* which the organisation faces in pursuing that strategy.

It is important to know what information the sponsors would request from the post holder, should they request any, and how frequently it would be required. Will the health authority or trust accept re-funding of the post if the sponsor withdraws? What controls are there to ensure that the agreed terms of the contract are not breached either by the sponsor placing covert pressure on the nurse to use more of its product or prescription service, or by the hospital manager accepting similar contracts with competitive manufacturers or soliciting bids from competitors for the sponsoring of the service?

The Future of Sponsorship

What of the long-term outcomes in health authorities accepting sponsorship of nursing roles? It is unlikely that only one or two companies will continue to offer some form of sponsorship if it is seen as a profitable initiative by competitive manufacturers. It is much more likely that other manufacturers, in varying specialty health care markets, will allocate a portion of their capital spending each year to such initiatives. It is quite feasible that if direct sponsorship of nursing roles continues, many senior nursing specialty posts around the country could be funded by individual sponsors.

As always, in a scenario such as this, there are positive and negative consequences of such actions to be considered. Many health authorities and trusts are hugely overspent. Their budgetary deficits often mean service rationalisation and possible cut-backs on non-essentials. If accepting an offer from a sponsor — any sponsor — means the funding of or continuation of one of the nursing posts under threat, the gain is measurable. Service to the patient can be assured and the post holder is made secure in her or his role for the duration of the term of agreement.

With such a 'grass roots' level of argument, does it really matter whether that service comes courtesy of an interested product manufacturer, as long as the service is there? Is there any problem in the majority of specialist nurses being funded in this way?

There are two arguments against this, the first being raised by Chadwick (1992), who writes:

> The argument against this is that, despite the apparent harmlessness of such arrangements, their increasing number reinforces the idea that health is not a public responsibility; that it is up to private concerns to finance it. In the long term it is difficult to see this as being in the interests of all, for a large concession is being made to the culture of publicity, which has been argued . . . to be an inappropriate one for the health service.

The second, and considerably stronger argument, considers the long-term changes wrought on the product industry and, ultimately, the quality of service received by the patient from an industry that now considers its primary market to be in the number of stoma care, continence advisory or breast care services it can fund, rather than its need to cater to the patient's changing world. Where is the justice in this for patients?

In this setting, long-term product development could be inhibited, and innovation curtailed as funding is redirected internally to finance the capital outlay required to sponsor a nursing role. The main casualty in this scenario is the patient. Could we still be claiming to serve our patients first in this setting, or would we be purely facilitating the increase of the annual net profit figure for companies getting rich on the backs of those needing health care services? These are not questions that are asked openly now, but they should perhaps be considered sooner or later.

When considering risk control systems in the light of

possible outcomes of sponsorship in nursing, these broader, ongoing issues of planning and funding of health care in the UK need to be handled at a much more senior level than that of hospital managers. These managers are trying to produce a working agreement that is fair to the sponsor and protective of the nurse's function, although the manager's input will indicate the local response to any negotiated agreement with a commercial sponsor and merits equal input from the specialist nurse involved.

Response by Professional Bodies and Support Agencies

When nurses, concerned by the emergence of this direct form of sponsorship, began to seek guidance and information, the obvious groups to turn to were the UKCC, the RCN and the RCN Stoma Care Nursing Forum. There were already in existence the UKCC guidelines in the form of the *Code of Professional Conduct* (1992).

In a separate statement on advertising and commercial sponsorship issued in 1991, the UKCC (1990) stated that:

> the Council has no basic objection to the devising and operation of schemes which raise additional funds to assist in diagnosis, treatment and care. It is concerned to ensure however, that income generating activities cannot damage the necessary relationship of trust between patients/clients and professional practitioners. Some commercial sponsorship plans that were suggested also caused concern.

The RCN Stoma Care Nursing Forum expressed its concern on behalf of its members in 1990 by putting forward the following resolution to Congress:

> That this meeting of the RCN Congress urges Council to examine the current position of health care agencies entering into sponsorship arrangements with private

companies and take appropriate action to persuade such
agencies to abandon these arrangements where the
independent judgement of nurses is compromised.

The resolution was supported by Congress, and subsequently two of the honorary officers of the Stoma Care
Nursing Forum met with officers and drew up guidelines
to assist members, whether managers or practitioners. The
guidelines were intended to help any nurse for whom
sponsorship might become an issue, but recognised that
stoma care nurses were, to date, the most likely to be
affected by this development.

The guidelines emphasised the importance of satisfac-
tory arrangements being made with the nurse, management and sponsor, and ethical and legal aspects were given
equal consideration. The guidelines were updated in April
1994 (RCN, 1994). They now provide a comprehensive
document detailing logical steps to be taken by all parties
involved in sponsorship agreements, and consider various
risk control mechanisms that may help to ensure both the
safety of the nurse's position, and the continued provision
of a fully impartial professional specialist nursing service
for the patient.

Other Interested Agencies

Although the inclusion of comments by other interested
agencies does not add directly to the ethical issues surrounding sponsorship in nursing, they are included here
because the positive and negative lessons to be learnt
regarding sponsorship in a health care setting are inextri-
cably linked with an appreciation of the business outcomes
of this type of arrangement.

The issue of sponsorship was raised as a concern by
some health service supply departments to the National

Audit Office in April 1991. It was pointed out that such deals involve NHS commitment to purchase specified quantities of products in return for the 'free' provision of associated or additional equipment or the funding of a nursing post. The report from the National Audit Office stated that these deals were open to objection on three main grounds:

- They are usually set up outside supplies controls, and are not necessarily subject to full commercial or financial evaluation.
- They bypass normal competitive tendering procedures.
- They subject NHS staff to pressures from suppliers (manufacturers). The National Audit Office concluded that NHS general managers should exercise strict control over such deals, and that any such deals should be subject to monitoring and appraisal to assess their net worth to the NHS.

In the autumn of 1991 an independent action group was formed, calling itself the Campaign For Impartial Stomacare. This group was chaired at the time by Ken Hargreaves, a former MP and himself an ileostomy patient. The aim of this group is stated to be:

> to look for ways to help nurses preserve their high standards
> of stomacare nursing in the United Kingdom and to act
> as a 'watchdog' organisation to investigate the area of
> company sponsorship in the stoma-care nursing field.

This group compiled a report for the benefit of the Department of Health on the issues of private funding of nursing posts. One of the recommendations of this report was that all sponsorship agreements should be passed through a local ethics committee for approval.

Conclusion

Some health authority managers responsible for accepting an offer of sponsorship have gone to great lengths to provide a deal which does not transgress professional responsibilities. Nurses providing a service that is funded by a commercial sponsor are aware of the need to provide and be seen to provide the most impartial of services. It may be that there is a degree of overreaction. As long as professional independence is maintained, should there be a more flexible attitude to sponsorship, both direct and indirect?

In order to adopt this argument, one would have to be aware of and comfortable with a series of safeguards ensuring that each party's rights were protected for the duration of the agreement. More importantly, one would need to be assured that the long-term consequences of this short-term initiative were to have no major negative implications for the specialist nursing roles, or for the patients who relied upon them. Are you assured?

References

Chadwick R (1992) Nursing advertising and sponsorship. In K Soothill, C Henry and K Kendrick (eds) *Themes and Perspectives in Nursing*. London: Chapman and Hall.

Gadow S (1980) Existential advocacy. In S F Spicker and G Gadow (eds) *Nursing Images and Ideals*. New York: Springer.

International Council of Nurses (1973) *Code for Nurses*. Geneva: ICN.

Johnson G and Scholes K (1989) *Exploring Corporate Strategy.* Hemel Hempstead: Prentice-Hall.

Kelly M P (1985) Loss and grief reactions as responses to surgery. *Journal of Advanced Nursing*, 10: pp. 517–25.

National Audit Office (1991) *National Health Service Supplies in England*. London: HMSO.

Orem D E (1985) *Nursing: Concepts of Practice* (3rd edn.). New York: McGraw Hill.

Royal College of Nursing (1994) Guidelines on Commercial Sponsorship of Nursing Posts, *Issues in Nursing and Health No. 9*. London: RCN.

Soloman R C and Hanson K R (1983) *Above the Bottom Line. An Introduction to Business Ethics*. New York: Harcourt Brace Jovanovich.

UKCC (1990) Registrar's letter, 3/1990, 23rd April 1990. London: UKCC.

UKCC (1992) *Code of Professional Conduct* (3rd edn.). London: UKCC.

Witts P (1992) Patient advocacy in nursing. In K Soothill, C Henry and K Kendrick (eds) *Themes and Perspectives in Nursing*. London: Chapman and Hall.

Index